the
make-up
book

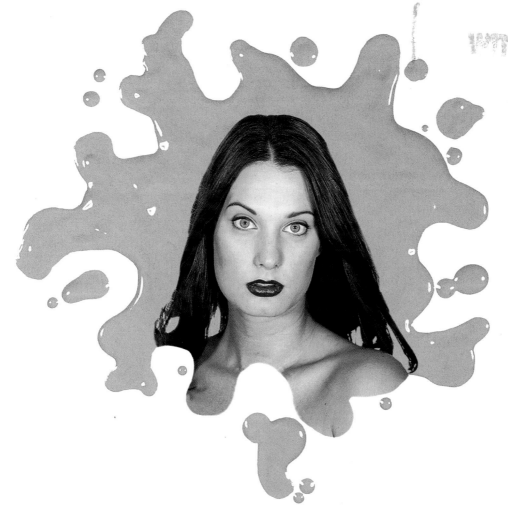

joy terri

NEW
HOLLAND

First published in 1999
by New Holland Publishers (UK) Ltd

London • Cape Town • Sydney • Auckland
www.newhollandpublishers.com

10 9 8 7 6 5 4 3

Garfield House
86-88 Edgware Road
London W2 2EA

80 McKenzie Street
Cape Town 8001
South Africa

Level 1, Unit 4
Suite 411, 14 Aquatic Drive
Frenchs Forest, NSW 2086
Australia

Unit 1A, 218 Lake Road
Northcote, Auckland
New Zealand

Publishing director: Linda de Villiers
Editor: Laura Milton
Design director: Janice Evans
Designer: Beverley Dodd
Make-up and styling: Joy Terri
Hairstylist: Donald Olive
Illustrator: Alix Korte

All photographs taken by Sean Waller, with the exception
of the following: cover front (bottom, far right), pages 28
(bottom right), 39 (bottom left and right), 46 (bottom
right), 67 (bottom left and right), 89 (second from the
bottom), 91, 92 (bottom left and right), 93 (top left and
right) and 94 (bottom left and right) by Henry Martin; and
pages 3 (third from the bottom), 6, 58 (bottom left), 67 (top),
87 (top row and bottom right) and 88 by Kelly Walsh.

Reproduction by Hirt & Carter Cape (Pty) Ltd
Printed and bound in Malaysia by Times Offset (M) Sdn Bhd

ISBN 1 85368 987 4 (hardcover)
ISBN 1 85974 099 5 (softcover)

author's acknowledgements

Very special thanks to my best friend and business partner, Debbie Jean, whose initial idea it was for me to write the book, and who motivated and supported me through it.

Thank you to my two very special make-up artists, Kerry Williams and Debbie Collins. Not only did you both give me moral support throughout working on the book, but also endless days of hard work. Your talents as make-up artists and models helped make this book possible.

An enormous thank you to Donald and the team at Sloanes Hair Company (especially Donovan) for your work on the hair in this book. Your excellent work motivated and assisted me and I couldn't have done it without you. I cannot think of better people to work with.

Thank you Sean Waller for the excellent photography. It was a great pleasure to work with you. Also thanks to both Kelly Walsh and Henry Martin for their photography.

And thank you, Alix, for your beautiful illustrations.

A special thank you to my editor, Laura, for your care, attention to detail and complete involvement in this book. I hope that we will be able to work together again in the future.

And special thanks to my designer, Bev, for your inspirational work that has made this book into what I wished it to be.

Thanks also to Linda and everyone else at Struik involved with producing the book.

I would also like to thank those who gave up their time to model for various sections in the book: Abeeda, Alayne, Alindi, Denise, Karen, Janice, Joanna, Jean, June, Lia, Lindy, Leander, Mom, Melanie, Sandy, Sibongele, Ying-Hung. Also, for your time, thanks to Wendy and Lindy W, Rosaline, Kim and Elanor.

Special thanks to André for all your love and patience. I couldn't have wished for better help and support during this time.

Thank you Duran and Rayne for your sacrifices throughout this book.

Thank you Mom and Dad for the love and support, as well as the enthusiasm you've shown for every project I've worked on. I thank you for where I am today and I hope to show my appreciation through making you as proud of me as I am of you.

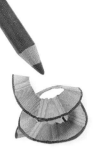

contents

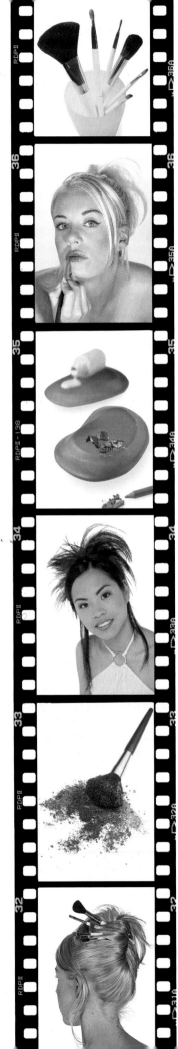

introduction

For years the art of applying make-up has been regarded as something mysterious taking place 'behind the scenes' in the fashion and film industry, with the magical 'tricks of the trade' applied to models and film stars only. The truth is that, with professional guidance, every woman can learn to use make-up to make the most of herself. In this book I would like to introduce some of the specialist products, tools and techniques that are at your disposal to help you create the exact effect you desire.

Make-up trends, like fashions in clothing, undergo constant change. Certain colours periodically gain popularity, as do certain styles. We are each offered a unique opportunity to respond – whether we accept, adapt or reject. Although many women will readily update their wardrobes to include something of the latest season's colours and styles, they are less likely to adapt their make-up to keep pace with changing trends and the development of new products. Some women only ever learn one way of applying make-up to their faces, and never stop to question what they are doing.

Women who 'decorate' their faces without questioning their technique often become so used to the 'decoration' that they begin relying on this look. They seldom, if ever, seek professional advice and never discover their true potential. If they do seek advice, they usually speak to a saleslady at a cosmetics counter who may also lack professional knowledge, and who may agree to almost anything that will help her sell her products.

Applied correctly, make-up can enhance a woman's beauty by accentuating striking features, or creating visual illusions, for example. A woman can use make-up to help her project an image of natural beauty, elegance or power, depending on what is appropriate. Applied incorrectly, however, make-up can actually detract from a woman's looks. A face may look different after make-up has been applied, but not necessarily better. A 'plain' face may merely be turned into a 'decorated' face, instead of a fresh-looking, elegant, or more youthful face.

Have you ever asked yourself whether you would allow anyone but a professional hairstylist to cut your hair? I do not not know any woman who would happily sport a noticeably 'amateur' haircut. When it comes to applying make-up, though, most women never consider that they may be creating a clearly 'amateur' look, and may even have been creating the same one for years.

The explanation may lie in the fact that make-up is so easy to remove. Imagine how much care we would take if we knew that, once applied, our make-up would be permanent, or even semi-permanent.

Not only do I love my work as a professional make-up artist, but I have also learned to make the most of my own looks. The self-confidence I have gained has made me a much happier, more positive and successful person, and I am passionate about sharing my knowledge with other women.

Everything you need to know has been brought together in this book, but, as in the case of any practical subject, you need to dedicate some time to learning the 'theory' and some time to practising the techniques described.

If you apply make-up at all, you will probably be applying it to your face for the rest of your life, so some hours spent practising now will prove to be a sound investment in your future.

As I said earlier, make-up trends change over the years, but the key to always looking your best lies in possessing knowledge of the winning combination of the correct make-up products, tools and professional techniques. Once you have gained this knowledge and mastered the various techniques, you will always be able to adapt your make-up look to being fashionable, whilst at the same time enhancing your particular features and making the most of your unique looks.

Joy Terri

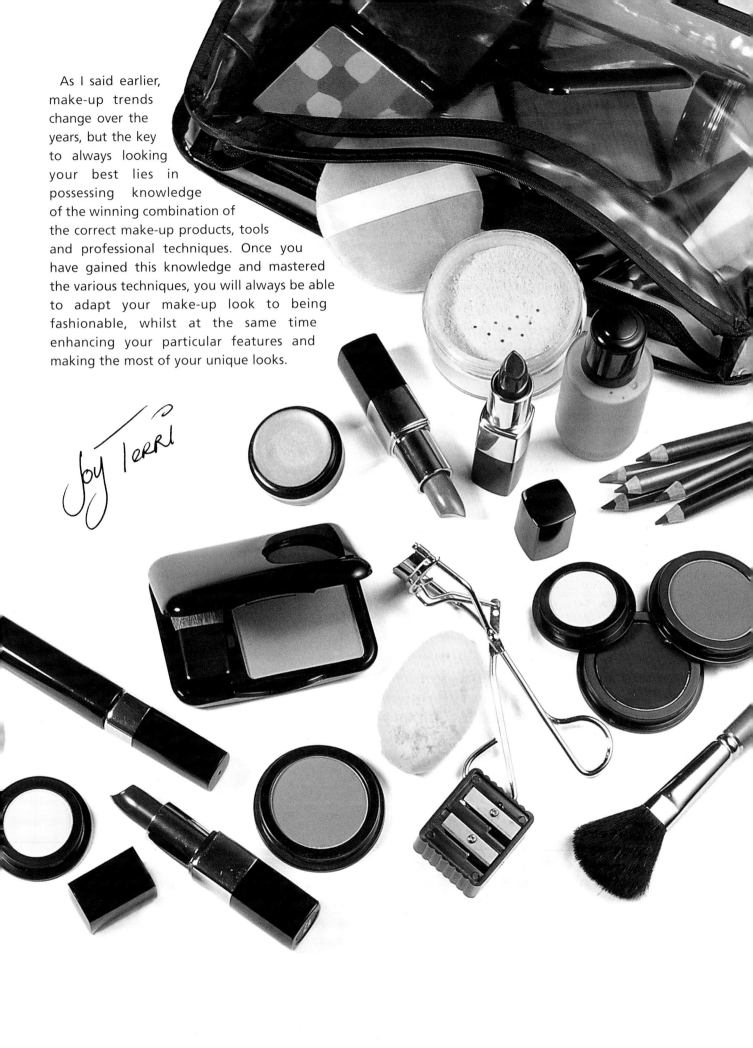

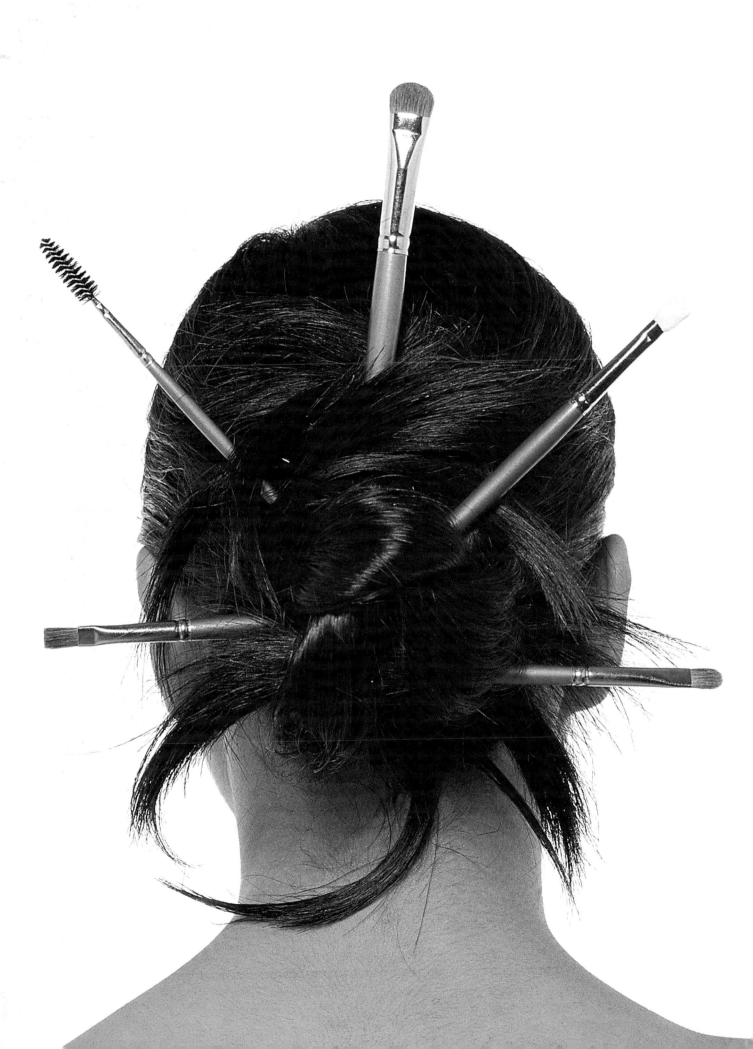

tools

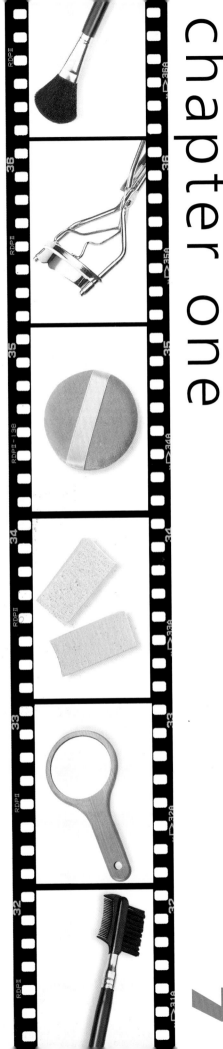

Quality make-up tools are an excellent investment – not meant only for use by professionals. If you are serious about looking your best at all times, and you are investing time in learning how experts in the field set to work, you also need to acquire the correct equipment. This chapter will show you what you need.

tools
of the trade

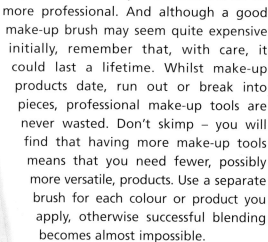

Many women will spend a fortune on make-up products, only to use inferior tools when it comes to applying those products to the skin. Avoid this costly mistake – pay as much attention to the applicator as to the product. It is no good using an excellent product, but botching the application because you lack the appropriate applicator. Once this is understood, it will be clear why I begin this book by addressing the choice of make-up tools.

Obtaining the correct applicators may seem like a daunting task at first, but, believe me, you will soon realize what a difference the right tools can make. Your make-up application will become quicker and easier, and the results you achieve will be far more professional. And although a good make-up brush may seem quite expensive initially, remember that, with care, it could last a lifetime. Whilst make-up products date, run out or break into pieces, professional make-up tools are never wasted. Don't skimp – you will find that having more make-up tools means that you need fewer, possibly more versatile, products. Use a separate brush for each colour or product you apply, otherwise successful blending becomes almost impossible.

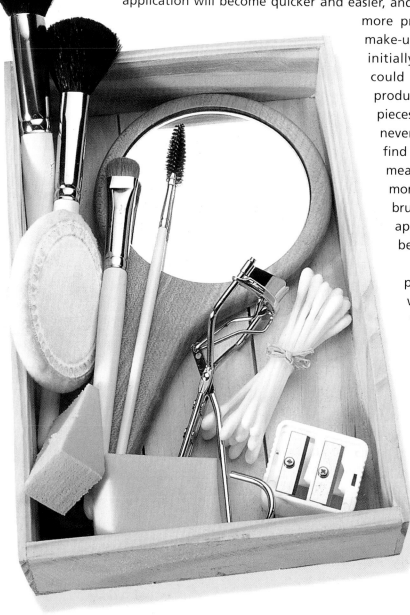

If possible, buy your tools from a professional make-up supplier. This will ensure quality, and save you from wasting money on expensive gimmicks. If you live far from a major centre, find out whether your nearest professional supplier is willing to mail your order to you (see page 95). All of the tools discussed on the pages that follow are available from professional make-up suppliers, and many of them are stocked by good department stores, pharmacies or health shops.

I recommend the following basic tools and accessories for your personal make-up kit.

general tools

a small sea sponge

A natural sea sponge, harvested when small, is soft and unabrasive. It is used for applying liquid foundation. Once wet, it has the advantage of not wasting the foundation by absorbing as much of it as a synthetic sponge would.

Wet the sponge thoroughly, squeeze out the water, then squeeze the sponge once more between the layers of a towel or in a tissue before using it to apply your foundation. Rinse it immediately after use.

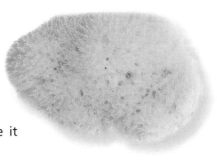

latex sponges

These sponges are extremely handy, as they can be used for various purposes, for example:

- in conjunction with a sea sponge to blend away edges or streaks of liquid foundation
- to apply powder or cream foundations
- to blend concealer.

Although latex sponges are available in different shapes and forms, the wedge shape is ideal for blending close to the eyelashes, as well as into the creases around the nostrils.

I prefer to work with these sponges when they are dry, but some make-up artists prefer to dampen the sponges first. Wash sponges once a week to keep them unclogged and free from grime, and replace a wedge as soon as it begins breaking up or changing texture.

powder puff

Use this puff to press powder onto your face. This procedure is the key to 'setting' your make-up. If you have been using a brush up until now, try a puff instead. You will notice a marked difference in terms of how long your make-up lasts, as a brush does not set the foundation in the same way as is done by using a patting action and a puff.

Good powder puffs are stitched together at the seams, not glued. They can easily be washed without coming apart.

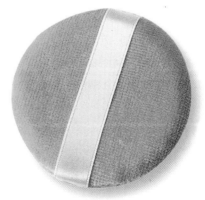

eyelash curler

This is a wonderful tool for those of us not blessed with lashes with a natural curl. It is not suggested that you use a curler every day – save it for special occasions.

tweezer

This is an essential tool for removing hair and maintaining a good eyebrow shape. Although tweezers are generally quite easy to find, it is worthwhile spending some time ensuring you find some that grip the hair really well. You may have to try out various brands.

sharpener

Sharp pencils are a must – for lips, eyes and brows. Invest in a versatile sharpener of good quality, and keep it clean.

handbag-sized shopping mirror

It is always a good idea to have this at the ready whenever you are shopping for make-up. It is next to impossible to test product colours inside stores using artificial light. If you have your own small mirror, you can walk to a source of natural light in the store and inspect the product you are testing on your face there. Make sure that your mirror is not too small – the mirrored section should not be smaller than the palm of your hand.

cotton buds & tissues

These disposable and inexpensive items come in handy at many different stages of make-up application. Cotton buds are ideal for blending make-up around the eye, and tissues are used to blot lipstick as well as to dust excess make-up off brushes during the process of application.

make-up brushes

powder brush

Use the largest brush in your kit as your powder brush. It should be soft and very smooth to the touch. First apply powder using a puff (see page 9), and then use this large brush to dust the excess powder from your face.

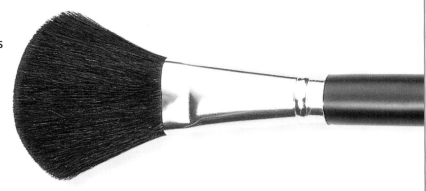

blusher brush

The best brush for applying blusher is more or less the size of the one pictured on the right. In addition to providing natural, healthy-looking colour, blusher is usually used to define the cheekbone and contour the face. If you use a larger brush, the blusher tends to colour too large an area of the cheek, or it creates an unflattering and obvious wide 'band' of colour. Using the correct brush will enable you to apply the colour far more precisely – both in terms of the amount of colour applied, as well as its position. Select a brush in which the brush hairs are not all cut to one length, but graduate gently, with shorter hairs on the outsides and longer hair at the centre. This will ensure an even distribution of blusher across the cheek, and help you avoid a 'patchy' look.

blusher blending brush

Your blending brush can be larger than your blusher brush and the hair can either be graduated or cut to one length. After applying blusher, the 'edges' of the line of colour are often too obvious, and so you need a clean brush to blend and soften the shape of the coloured area. This brush should never be dipped into the container of your blusher so that it becomes coated with blusher itself. It should always be kept clean and only be used for blending.

dome-shaped eye-shadow brushes

Small, dome-shaped brushes are used for applying eye shadows. A separate brush must be used for each colour of shadow used, for instance one for shading and one for highlighting. In brushes of this shape, the hair is graduated from short to long in a rounded, dome shape. As the hairs do not end in a straight line, the particles of eye-shadow powder cling to the brush evenly along the shaped part.

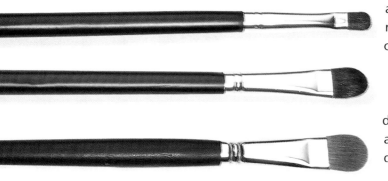

When the brush touches the skin, therefore, the powder is not all deposited in one patch. The brush allows the particles of shadow to be distributed evenly across the eyelid.

Dome-shaped brushes are available in different sizes. Larger brushes are used to shade larger areas on the eye, and smaller brushes for smaller areas. The best small brushes are made of sable hair – this is smooth and soft, and does not pull or tug at the skin in the delicate eye area. Your smallest brush should be soft, yet firm enough to enable you to apply eye shadow close to the upper and lower lashes in a neat, thin line. This is useful when lining the eyes with dark eye shadow (see page 69), rather than using pencil eyeliner.

flat eye-shadow brush

This flat brush with the hair tips ending in a straight line is used to blend away hard edges of eye-shadow colour. As is the case with a brush used to blend blusher, this brush should not be dipped into the powder container at all, but be kept clean and used only for blending away hard lines.

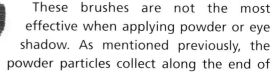

These brushes are not the most effective when applying powder or eye shadow. As mentioned previously, the powder particles collect along the end of the hair in a straight line and, when applied to the skin, there is not a gradual distribution of colour. Often a 'blotch' of shadow is deposited where all the powder lands as the brush touches the skin.

Straight-edged, flat brushes should never be 'dipped' into eye shadow or blusher in a container (see page 64). They tend to hit the product with more force than a dome-shaped brush. This often leads to compacted powder products breaking up into pieces, and much of the product thus being wasted.

liquid eyeliner brush

If you use liquid eyeliner often, it is worthwhile investing in one of these brushes. It makes the application so much easier. This professional brush designed specifically for lining eyes is made of sable hair which graduates towards a clean point. You

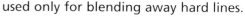

will be able to apply a clean, neat line, without the hair separating.

eyebrow brush, eyelash comb & mascara wand

The little brush shown here is used to brush eyebrows up and outwards to create a neat shape. Apply mascara using the appropriate wand and, if necessary, use the small comb to comb the mascara through the lashes evenly, removing any 'blobs'. Many make-up artists also use a wand-type applicator for brushing eyebrows effectively.

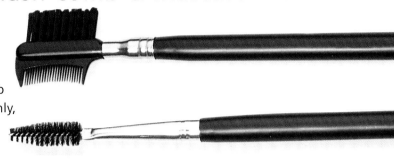

angled eyebrow brush

This is used instead of or with an eyebrow pencil to apply shadow to the eyebrows, to darken them or to fill in spaces created by uneven hair growth. The slanted shape is ideal for creating the illusion of small, slanting eyebrow hairs in between existing ones.

   The brush shown here is made of hog hair, but similar brushes are available made from sable hair. If your eyebrow hair is fine, choose sable hair; if your eyebrow hair is coarse, choose a brush made of hog hair.

lipstick brush

As lipstick is such a sticky substance, a firm brush is required for its successful application. Brushes made of sable hair are generally best for working the lipstick onto your lips. Some make-up artists prefer working with quite small lipstick brushes to ensure a clean lip edge, however, as clean an edge can be achieved using an average-sized brush carefully.

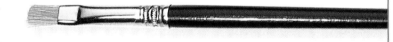

concealer brush

Concealer is also a sticky substance like lipstick, so once again a small sable hair brush is ideal. For concealing blemishes, a brush with a very fine tip is necessary so that only a tiny dot of concealer can be applied at a time. The aim is to cover the blemish alone – not the surrounding area.

fan brush

This brush is an optional extra, used for dusting off loose powder. Its shape is ideal for sweeping excess powder away from the eye area. It can also reach into the creases at the sides of the nose.

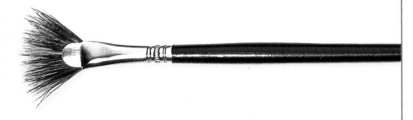

natural or synthetic hair?

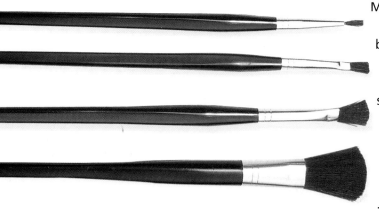

Manufacturers of make-up brushes have realized that women often purchase brushes or commercial brush kits because they look colourful and attractive, rather than because of their particular shape, size or texture. This has meant that simple, good make-up brushes have become quite hard to find. Colourful brushes in pretty pots that match the colour scheme of your bedroom may look nice, but often very little thought has gone into the real purpose of the brushes.

Cheap, colourful brushes are often made using synthetic hair, which is coarse and scratchy. These brushes damage make-up products in compacted powder form, as they quickly break them up into dust, and the brush hairs have rarely been cut into the correct domed shape to apply make-up successfully. The hair of synthetic brushes also often loses its shape quite soon. The brush too easily flares into a 'fountain' shape, making application rather difficult and messy.

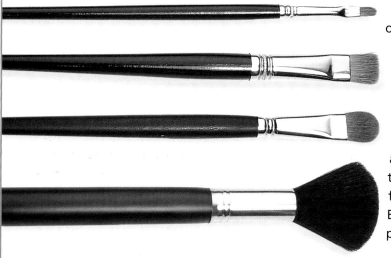

Professional make-up brushes are made of natural animal hair. Depending on the flexibility requirements of the brush, a particular choice of hair is made. For eye-shadow brushes, sable hair is the most suitable, although it may also be the most expensive. Sable hair is soft, smooth and gentle on the delicate skin around the eye. At the same time, it has the correct degree of firmness required for effective make-up application. Brushes for applying blusher and powder are made of softer natural hair.

Professional brushes made of natural hair are also very carefully cut into shapes designed for particular purposes. Make-up application becomes neater, easier and quicker. In addition, used correctly, brushes made of natural hair do not damage compact eye shadows and blushers as much as synthetic brushes, so you will find that your make-up products last far longer.

Brushes made of natural hair may seem expensive initially, but they are made to last. They save you constantly having to replace brushes, or products that have been broken into bits by coarse and scratchy synthetic brushes.

cleaning your brushes

All your make-up brushes should be cleaned at least once a month. Brushes used to apply lipstick and concealer require more frequent cleaning than brushes used for powder products, though, as these brushes often become sticky and then easily pick up particles of dust and dirt.

Brushes can be washed in warm water with pure soap or mild hair shampoo. Make sure that you wash brushes gently, retaining the shape of the brush hair and not flaring it out into a fountain shape. Gently squeeze out the make-up while the brush is under the water. Follow the same procedure and rinse brushes thoroughly in clean water, ensuring that all traces of soapiness have been removed. Squeeze the hair back into its original shape and place the brushes on a clean, dry towel to dry.

Make-up brushes may also be cleaned without water, just by using certain quite strong chemicals. Until recently these chemicals have only been available professionally, owing to their toxicity and danger in the home environment. Some manufacturers have now come up with non-toxic formulas, though, and these can be ordered from professional make-up suppliers. You simply dip your brushes into the cleaner, remove them and wipe them on a tissue. They are dry almost immediately, as the cleaner evaporates instantly. It only takes seconds to completely remove even sticky red lipstick from your brush.

space & light

It is important to create a comfortable space for everyday make-up application. There is no point investing in tools and products, and learning professional techniques if you are going to try to apply your make-up using the rear-view mirror of your car on your way to work every day, for example.

Firstly, you need sufficient space to set out your make-up kit in front of you. As make-up containers are generally difficult to keep clean, it may be a good idea to get into the habit of unpacking all the products you need, and opening all the lids before you begin applying anything. When you have completed your application, wash or wipe your fingers, close all the containers, and return them to your make-up bag. You will find that the containers and the bag stay remarkably clean.

When applying make-up, it is essential that light is distributed evenly over your face. Always use a cool lamp, and one that emits light which is as close as possible in colour to natural daylight. Normal household globes emit considerable heat and create a yellow glow that can be quite misleading when you select make-up colours.

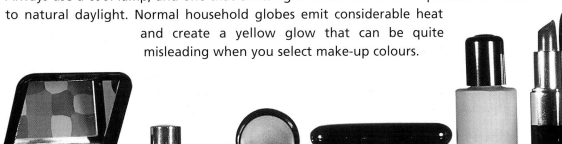

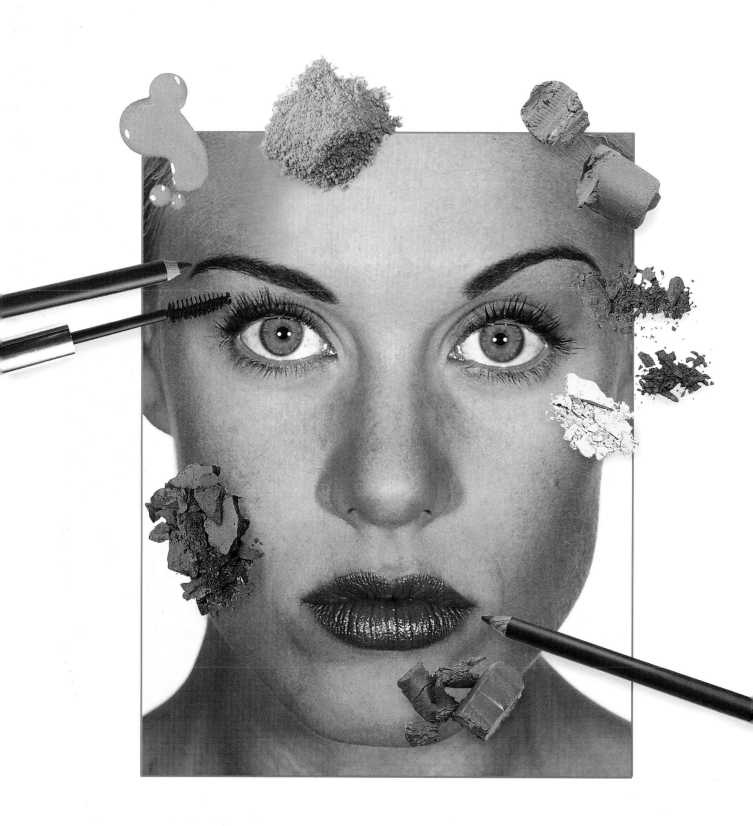

products

chapter two

To achieve a truly professional make-up

finish you not only require the correct

tools, but also the correct make-up

products. So as not to be overwhelmed

by the array of products facing you, it is

essential to have a clear understanding

of the functions of each product.

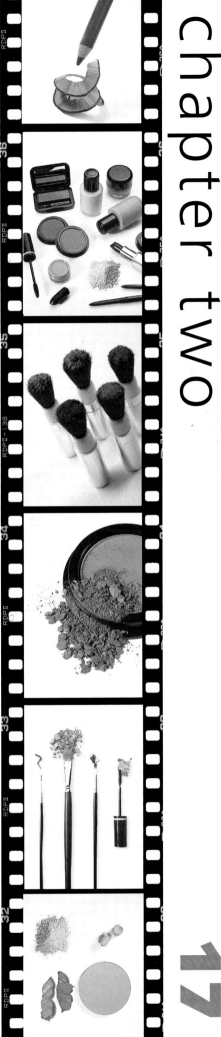

basic
explanations

In my view it is of great importance to have a clear understanding the function of each make-up product used during the application process. This will enable you to identify exactly what you need, and to shop accordingly. You will also know what the specific product should be able to accomplish for you, and what you can and cannot expect from it. Testers at make-up counters not only allow you to test the *colour* of a product on your skin, but also to judge its *quality and texture* in terms of the particular function you require it to perform.

There should, for example, be a distinct difference in texture between a pencil used for eyebrows, and one used as an eyeliner. Knowing what to look for – and not simply reading the manufacturer's label on the pencil – is what counts. The same goes for other make-up products and, if you are not satisfied with what you find in the shops, you can always contact a professional make-up supplier (see page 95).

This chapter gives an overview of the basic products used to put together a good make-up kit. Once you have a good grasp of the function of each product, and are aware of what is available, you will be able to make an informed choice about which type of product you require.

foundation

Foundation products are used to create an even skin tone, and to smooth the skin texture to create a seemingly flawless finish. Foundation is meant to provide light to medium coverage, not to cover pigmentation marks, blemishes, dark rings under the eyes and so forth – this is why you may require a separate concealer.

Foundation also provides a base for the subsequent application of other make-up products Eye shadows, blushers and lipsticks, for instance, are not designed for use on skin without foundation. In fact, if you add colours to the 'naked' face without using foundation, the make-up colour you add will exaggerate the unevenness in the skin tone and could result in blemishes and flaws being more noticeable. In addition, other products will not blend or last as well on skin without foundation.

Quite possibly nothing is more important than finding (or mixing) foundation to match your skin colour exactly. A 'close' match is simply not good enough – it has to be exact and 'invisible' once applied.

Nowadays a vast range of foundation products is available. Textures vary enormously, in addition to being water-based, oil-based or oil-free, and consistency and coverage differ greatly. Most good make-up houses offer a wide range of colours to match your skin tone. Take time to experiment – it is your right be assertive and to insist on testing and comparing various brands. Foundation usually takes one of three basic forms: liquid, cream, or powder.

liquid foundation

Liquids generally offer light to medium coverage, but the precise extent of coverage depends on the particular brand and on how thickly the liquid is applied.

Liquid foundations offer the widest range of colours, and if you are unable to find an exact match to your skin tone, colours can be mixed to obtain an in-between shade. Do not mix foundations of different brands, though. Keep to products of the same kind from a single make-up house. If you have never used foundation, there is no need to be concerned that your face will look unnaturally 'painted'. If foundation is matched to the skin tone exactly, a wonderfully natural appearance can be achieved.

For very dry skin, choose an oil-based foundation. For normal skin, choose a water-based foundation, and for very oily skin, choose foundation labelled 'oil-free'.

cream foundation

A cream that feels slightly dry to the touch will usually offer light to medium cover. Very rich, often stodgy creams offer medium to heavy cover, and are used mostly for stage and film make-up. These heavier creams are not suggested for use on mature skin.

powder foundation

This type of foundation was developed more recently than liquid or cream foundations. It has been designed for women who need to apply their make-up in a hurry or for those who dislike the feel of liquid or cream foundation on the skin.

Powder foundation can be understood as two products combined into one – foundation and powder. When using other types of foundation, the subsequent application of powder is required to 'set' the foundation. If you use a powder foundation, however, you can omit a separate, subsequent application of powder.

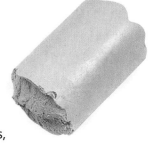

concealer

This product is applied to provide extra cover to specific areas where foundation has not been sufficient to create an even skin tone. It may be used to conceal blemishes, dark rings under the eyes, or unwanted redness still obvious on the cheeks, nose or chin, for example.

In addition, concealer applied to the entire eyelid provides a wonderful base for eye shadow, helping it to blend easily and last throughout the day without settling into the creases of the eyes.

It is important that your concealer is one or two shades lighter in colour than your foundation, but that it has the same undertone. For example, if your foundation is beige with a yellowish undertone, then your concealer should also have a yellowish undertone, and not a pinkish one.

Concealer is available in several forms: mainly as a liquid, as a stick, and as a cream.

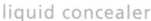

liquid concealer

The packaging of this form of concealer often contains a wand applicator. The advantage of a liquid is that it blends softly and easily without you having to tug at the skin. While being useful for concealing pigmentation on the eyelids, for instance, this kind of concealer does not offer enough cover to mask blemishes.

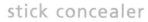

stick concealer

This form of concealer generally offers good cover for blemishes. It may be difficult to blend without pulling the skin, however, so avoid using it around the delicate eye area.

cream concealer

This concealer, often packaged in a small tub, is the form of concealer most commonly used by make-up artists because it has the perfect consistency. Cream concealers have the advantages of both the liquid and stick forms, without any of the disadvantages. The cream is sticky enough to cling to areas that require cover, while also being soft enough to blend easily. It is good for concealing blemishes, dark rings under the eyes, or undesirable red tinges still showing through the foundation. It is also soft and comfortable enough to use around the eye area without stretching the skin during application.

powder

There are several very good reasons for using powder. Most importantly, powder 'sets' your foundation and makes it last. It also adds a matte finish that always looks fresh, professional, and chic. Powder can make the skin texture seem finer, as it makes the pores look smaller. Lastly, powder removes any stickiness created by foundation or concealer. After powdering, eye shadow or blusher can be applied and blended easily on a silky smooth skin.

It is very important to ensure that the powder you use does not change the colour of your foundation. If you have succeeded in matching your foundation to your skin colour perfectly, you do not want to change it now by applying powder that contains too much colour, especially not pink.

Powder is generally available in loose, translucent form or in pressed form.

loose, translucent powder

Most of the loose powders offered by make-up houses are not translucent in the true sense of the word, as they inevitably contain a certain amount of colour. In addition, there are usually only a few shades to choose from. Therefore, most make-up artists prefer using professional translucent powder that does not contain any real colouring. By so doing they do not risk changing the foundation colour already carefully matched to the skin.

Loose powder does not build up on the skin and create a heavy, caked look. It is extremely light and if too much is applied, the excess can easily be dusted off with a large, soft brush.

pressed powder

The one distinct advantage of pressed powder is that it is much less messy to carry in your handbag than loose powder. For this reason, it can sometimes be handy for quick touch-ups during the course of the day. You also generally have a wider range of shades to choose from than in the case of loose powder. If you opt for pressed powder, find a shade as close as possible to the colour of your foundation, and only use it sparingly. The disadvantage of pressed powder is that it tends to build up on the skin if applied repeatedly, and one needs to be aware of this when doing touch-ups.

yellow colour correctors

The majority of women have yellowy skin tones, rather than pink skin tones. Make-up houses have overlooked this fact for years, and many of them have been manufacturing foundations, concealers and powders containing far too much pink colouring for their make-up products to look completely natural. The aim of foundations, concealers and powders is to make skin seem flawless. If the products applied differ from the natural skin colour, though, a really natural look with 'invisible' make-up cannot be achieved.

Some make-up houses have begun to realize that they need to improve their colour ranges, and they are beginning to produce products with yellower tones, as well as yellow colour correctors to be mixed with their other products. If these correctors are not yet freely available in your part of the world, contact a professional make-up supplier (see page 95) and you may arrange a mail order.

Yellow powder is a translucent powder with an added yellow colouring. It can be used to create a finish as close as possible to one's natural skin tone. As a make-up artist, I use yellow powder on women with all skin tones, with the exception of those who are very fair.

To match certain skin tones I find that, in addition to using yellow powder, I also need to add a yellow base to the foundation to achieve a perfect match. Add as little or as much corrector as you need to match your skin.

eyebrow pencil

This kind of pencil is used to define and darken the eyebrows, or to pencil them in, and to create the illusion of even hair growth throughout the length of the brow. A good eyebrow pencil needs to be hard and dry, so that you can draw crisp, clean lines, and not create smudgy brows that look painted. Many pencils that are labelled 'eyebrow pencil' are far too soft to create the desired effect. Before buying, test the texture of the pencil by drawing on the back of your hand – the line should be crisp.

In terms of colour, eyebrow pencils are generally available in black, dark brown, light brown and grey. If you choose a light brown colour, take care not to choose one with a strong rusty tinge to it – this colour almost always looks 'false' unless you are a true fiery redhead. If you are very fair, it is safest to choose a pale ash-brown colour.

eyebrow shadow

This is used instead of pencil or sometimes applied over eyebrow pencil to create a natural finish. It can only be used as a pencil substitute where there is substantial hair growth. In fact, many make-up artists actually prefer using shadow to pencil in the latter case. Eyebrow shadow alone should not be used where hair growth is very sparse.

eye shadow

Make-up in the form of eye shadow is used around the eyes to draw attention to them and to enhance their natural shape. Eye shadow is available in pressed and loose powder forms, as well as in cream forms, and in matte, frosted or iridescent formulas. It is probably most widely available in pressed powder form, and the range of colours and shades is vast. On pages 48–57 colours have been categorized to guide you in selecting which are suitable.

As a general rule I recommend that you have three shades of eye shadow to work with during a single application:

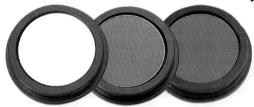

◆ a light colour (white, for example), referred to as your *highlighter*

◆ a medium or darkish shade (medium brown, for example), referred to as your *shading colour*

◆ a very dark shade (dark brown/black, for example), referred to as your *framing colour*.

eyeliner

This is used to create a darkened frame around each eye, drawing attention to the eyes and accentuating their beauty. Eyeliner can also be used to create illusions around the eyes, making them appear larger, or more elongated, for example.

It is very important that you always choose pencil eyeliners that are very soft, so that shading can gently and easily be applied to the delicate skin around the eye. Pencils used on this area should not scratch or tug at the skin, thereby stretching it. The shading should blend easily if you want to soften the line with a cotton bud. Test pencils before buying by drawing on your hand and then smudging the line gently. Pencil eyeliners are available in assorted colours, but for equipping an everyday make-up kit I recommend dark brown and/or black.

Not only pencils are used to outline eyes, though, as many make-up artists prefer using very dark eye shadow. Some never use a pencil at all, because shadow is softer on the skin and looks more natural than a hard, pencilled line. The quality of eye shadow used is important, though, as you should be able to apply it neatly without messing. Shadow will also last longer around the eye than pencil.

I do not recommend liquid eyeliner for everyday use, as it can so easily look messy if not applied correctly. I have therefore discussed it separately on page 25.

mascara

This is used to thicken and darken the eyelashes which, in turn, enhance the beauty of the eyes. Mascara is generally available in dark brown, black and charcoal grey, as well as in various consistencies in regular and waterproof formulas. Although it is also available in navy, blue, and a number of other colours, these are fashion fads. Do not make a habit of using them regularly. And remember, if you use waterproof mascara, you will need an appropriate remover.

blusher

The function of blusher is either to define the cheekbone or to soften a cheekbone that is too prominent, and to enhance and contour the shape of the face. Blusher can also be used to add natural colour to the face. These aspects are discussed in detail on pages 74–77.

Blushers are available in pressed powder and cream forms. Whichever form you choose, keep to natural colours with a matte finish. Never choose a bright pink or a bright orange blusher. This will defeat the purpose of the application.

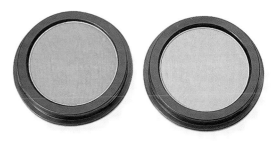

lip pencil

Lips are outlined to define the mouth and create a clean, neat border for lipstick application. Lip liners can also be used to correct the shape of the lips if they are unbalanced, for instance, by enlarging a top lip slightly. This is much easier to accomplish when using a lip pencil than it is when using lipstick alone (see pages 81–83).

When choosing a lip pencil, test the quality on the back of your hand. It should not be soft and smudgy. Lip pencils are made with less oil and from a much harder wax than lipstick. This is done so that your lip outline will last, and not 'bleed' beyond the lip edge the way lipstick can. Lip liners are available in a variety of colours and should be matched as closely as possible to your lipstick colour.

lipstick

A neat application of a suitable lipstick adds finish to a look and colour to the face. In addition, it draws attention to your lips, and to your smile. Most lipsticks sold at cosmetics counters are presented in a stick form.

Lipsticks are available in cream and frosted formulas, and in a wide variety of colours. Some offer a high degree of coverage and the appearance of solid colour, while others are more sheer, working with the natural lip colour. Some formulas have been designed to last through several hours of wear without requiring reapplication. When buying lipstick, test various colours and textures, as some may feel very dry on the lips. Then choose the formula you find most comfortable to wear.

optional extras

As technology develops, new or improved 'problem-solving' products are constantly appearing on the shelves. These are not essentials, but can be exceptionally useful.

anti-shine

This is a great product for applying to oily skins or oily T-panels. It is generally applied before foundation, and immediately creates a matte effect. The skin is also kept matte for far longer periods than can be achieved by using powder. You may not readily find this product at your local beauty counter, but it can usually be obtained from a professional make-up supplier (see page 95).

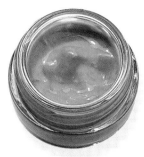

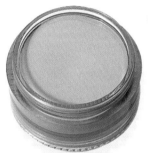

green colour corrector

The most commonly used colour corrector is green. It functions in a similar way to concealer, but the green colour is far more effective in counteracting redness in the skin, as in the case of blemishes, broken veins, or very ruddy cheeks, for example. Your usual concealer is then applied over the colour corrector.

liquid eyeliner

This product can be used instead of pencil eyeliner, but on the top lid only. A liquid eyeliner creates a much stronger, more definite line, but should preferably be kept for dramatic evening applications and then used only if you can achieve a very straight, clean line (see page 70).

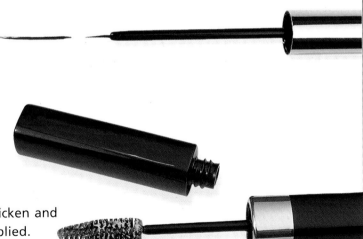

eyelash thickener

This almost transparent coating is used to thicken and lengthen the eyelashes before mascara is applied.

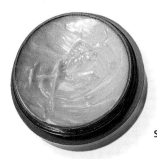

lip gloss

To add extra shine to your lips, use lip gloss. It is available in tinted or colourless formulations and can be used alone or over lipstick. It is not recommended for use on mature skin, as it tends to 'bleed' into any little lines around the lips.

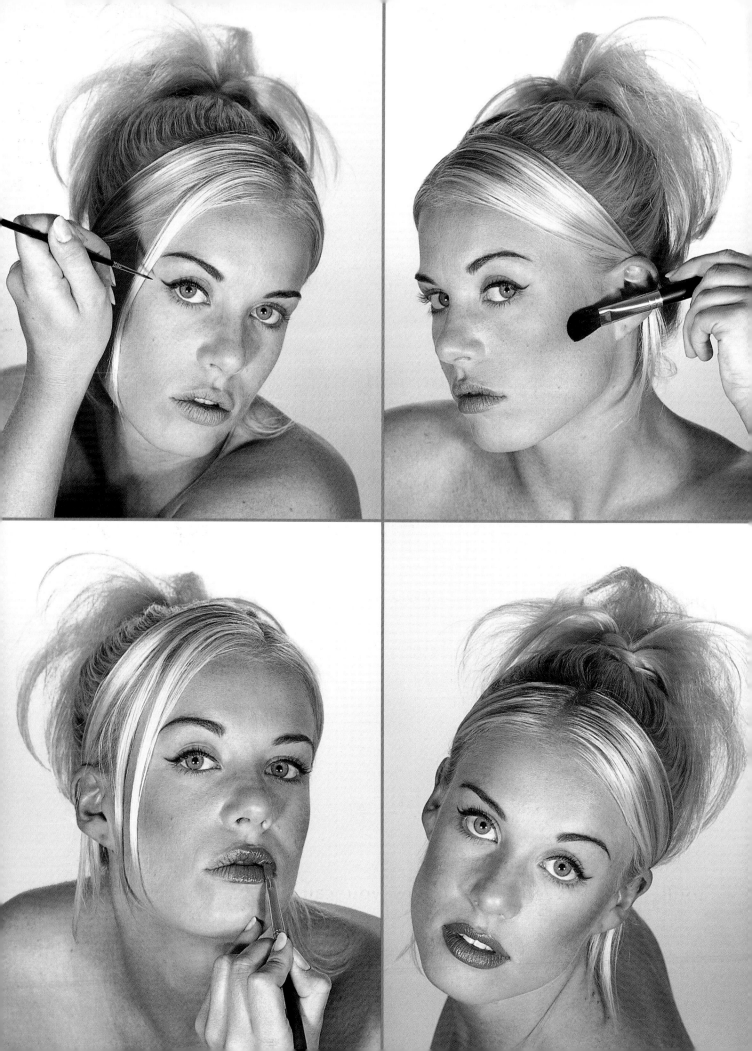

techniques

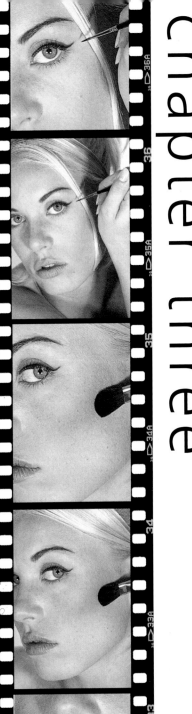

Once you have discovered which make-up tools to use, and understand how each make-up product functions, you can move on to mastering various make-up techniques. By combining the correct tools, products and techniques you can create any look you desire.

eyebrows
shape up

Make-up artists regard eyebrows as the most important feature of a woman's face. If your eyebrows are shapeless and untidy, they can ruin any make-up effect you try to create. If you have been neglecting your eyebrows – not realizing their significance – study this section carefully, paying particular attention to the instant 'eye-lift' illusion which is illustrated below.

The aim of removing hair from the eyebrow area is not only to thin out and neaten brows, but also to create a shape that enhances the eye. Many women pluck their eyebrows, but do not achieve a shape allowing them to create balance and illusion around the eye. Make sure that you have a clear idea of the shape you wish to achieve by studying all the photographs and illustrations in this section. Only then pick up a pair of tweezers.

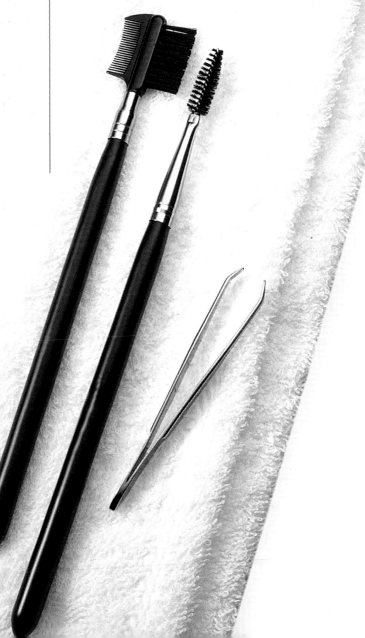

the 'eye-lift' illusion

In the photograph below the eyebrow on the right has been carefully plucked to create a beautiful, arched shape. The eyebrow on the left has been left in its natural state. Look at the illusion of 'lift' created on the side of the face where the eyebrow has been shaped. The area above the eye has been opened up, providing a clear space above the lid to be shadowed cleverly, and a face that will look much more elegantly finished.

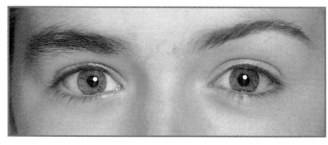

If you want to make the most of your looks, do not neglect your eyebrows. Look at the illusion of 'lift' created by removing hair from the eyebrow on the right.

the ideal eyebrow shape

As a guide to achieving the ideal eyebrow shape, look at the photograph below, and imagine similar lines being drawn across your own face.

A The thickest part – where the eyebrow begins – should be close to a point on a vertical line running roughly from the outside of the nose up towards the forehead.

B The outside of the eyebrow should end at a point on a line running from the corner of the nose past the outer corner of the eye.

C If you divide the length of the eyebrow into three equal sections, the highest point of the arched shape should be approximately two thirds outwards from the starting point.

Note that the eyebrow shape stretches up and outwards in a straight line and thins out on its decline. Any hair growing outside this desired shape is removed. It is a good idea to use a dark eyebrow pencil to practise drawing this shape over or through your brows as they currently are. If you find yourself having drawn an unsatisfactory shape, clean off the pencilled markings and start afresh. Make sure that you have achieved two more or less equal, balanced brow shapes (i.e. so that your two eyebrows match each other as closely as possible in shape) before you begin removing any hair.

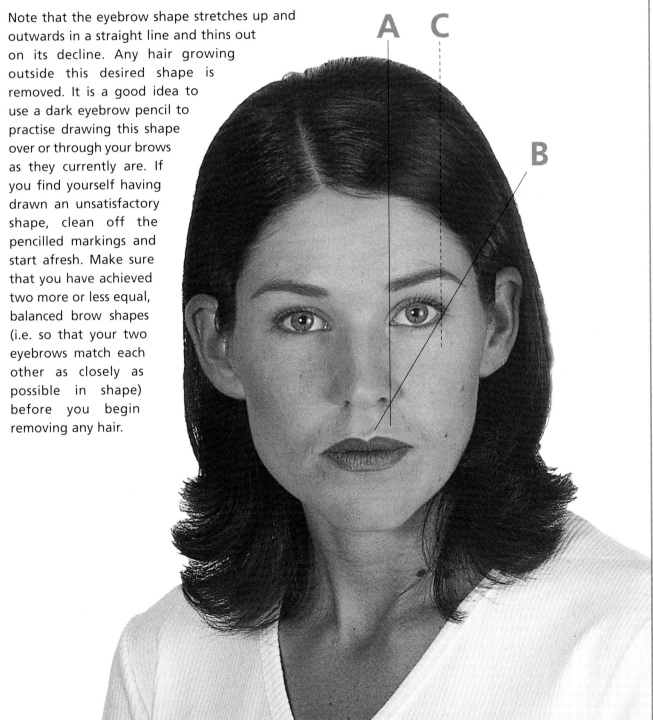

where to begin

Some women have been taught that only the outsides of the eyebrows (i.e. the area furthest from the nose) should be plucked to create an arch. They have been told that the start of the eyebrow (i.e. closest to the nose) should never be touched. Used on thick, heavy eyebrows, however, this practice will result in an unbalanced eyebrow shape. The start of the eyebrow will seem too heavy, and the shape will not create the desired illusion of 'lift' around the eye. This is a common mistake made when plucking to remove hair, so examine the diagrams below carefully.

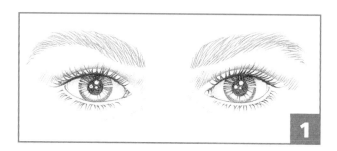

1 Here are the eyebrows in their natural state, before any hair has been removed.

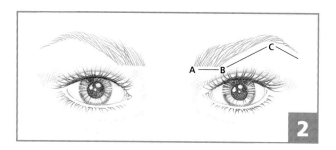

2 The eyebrows have only been thinned along the outsides. This has resulted in unbalanced brows with too much heaviness remaining close to the nose. Note the straight line from A to B, and the short upward slant from B to C. Not much illusion of 'opening' and 'lifting' has been created.

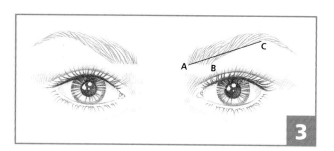

3 By connecting points A and C with a straight line and removing the hair below the line at corner B, a significant improvement can be achieved. Note how a much longer upward slant is achieved with the creation of one unbroken line stretching from A to C.

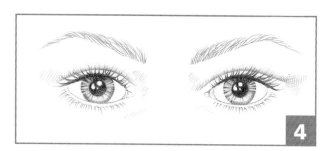

4 This is the final shape to be aimed for. Significantly more space has been opened up between the eye and the eyebrow, creating the desired illusion of 'lift'. The shape of the eyebrow now consists of one long, unbroken line stretching up to the peak, and then gently sloping down.

thinly plucked eyebrows

If you are already in the habit of plucking your eyebrows quite thinly, or if your eyebrows are naturally thin, you may still be able to improve on their shape by plucking.

1 The first photograph shows eyebrows that have already been plucked thinly. A better shape can still achieved, however, by further shaping at the start of the eyebrow (as indicated in the illustrations opposite).

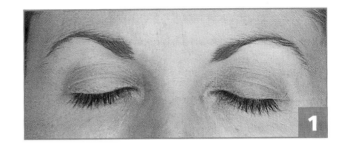

2 This photograph shows just a small amount of hair having been removed. The eyebrow shape is more balanced and the effect is far more professional.

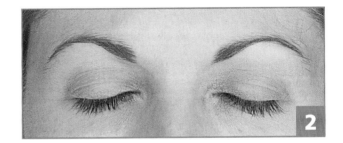

3 The final photograph shows the elegant new shape created once the eyebrows are defined with a little dark brown shadow.

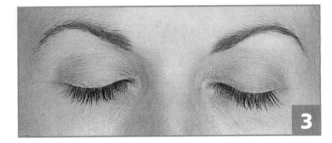

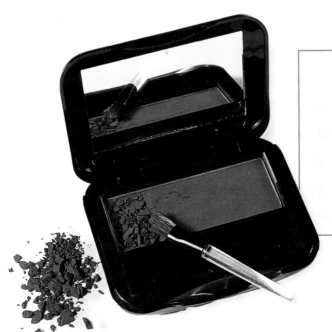

Do not judge the look of your brows when you have just plucked them, and not yet defined them. Once you have defined them with dark shadow, you will have a far better idea of the finished effect.

how to pluck

Always bear in mind that no-one has two perfectly symmetrical eyebrows. You will have to work with the natural hair growth of each brow in turn, achieving as symmetrical and even a look as possible. Defining brows with shadow or pencil after plucking can create the illusion of symmetry.

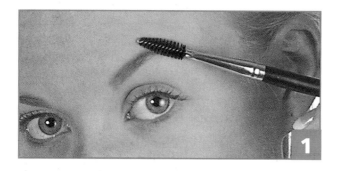

1 Using an eyebrow brush or a mascara wand, brush all the eyebrow hair on both eyebrows diagonally upwards.

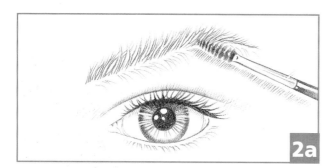

2a Now you can 'part' the brow hair as shown, brushing the hair to be removed downwards. The hair brushed upwards will not be plucked, and will form the final desired shape.

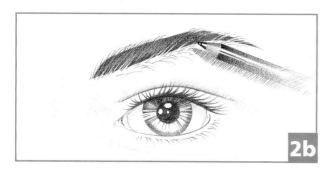

2b Alternatively, you can use a dark eyebrow pencil, or even a black eyeliner pencil, to draw in the desired eyebrow shape through the existing hair. Exaggerate the shading considerably, so that the desired shape is clearly visible. Any hair outside the shaded area will then be removed.

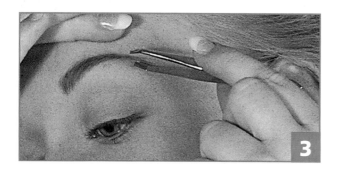

3 You now need to remove the unwanted hair. Hold the tweezers in one hand, and use the other hand to lightly stretch the skin of the area you are about to tweeze. Grasp each hair as close to its root as possible, and pluck in the direction of the natural hair growth. Work carefully, ensuring that you do not remove hair unnecessarily.

uneven eyebrows

It is normal to have uneven hair growth along the length of the eyebrow. There may be patches where hair growth is sparse, and patches where the hair is thicker. You may also, for instance, have thick, full brows at the start, and almost no hair where the brow ends towards the temples.

When it comes to applying your make-up, either an eyebrow pencil or shadow may be used to even out the appearance of brows. This technique is explained and illustrated on pages 44–47.

1 These uneven eyebrows have not yet been shaped.

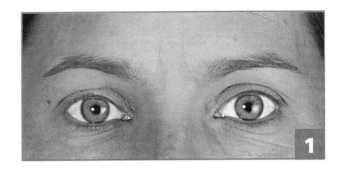

2 Now unwanted hair has been removed and the desired shape has been created.

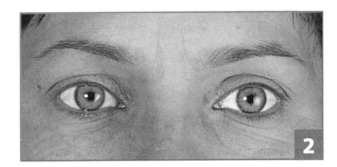

3 The final result is achieved by subtly shading the brows to provide definition and a neat, elegant finish. Note how any uneven patches have been filled in.

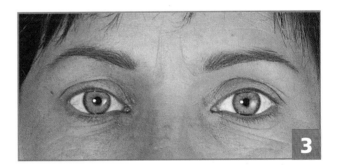

If you prefer visiting a beauty salon, make sure that the beauty therapist has a clear idea of what you want. You may wish to pencil in the desired eyebrow shape yourself, and ask for only the hair outside this shape to be removed, or take this book along as a guide to explaining the shape.

foundation, concealer & powder
create the base

Every woman I know would love to have perfect skin, but for the vast majority of us this is an impossible dream. Even the most beautiful models that appear in glossy magazines have 'imperfections' that require concealing, or have their photographs retouched before publication.

By learning the art of correctly applying foundation, concealer and powder, however, many women will find it possible to create the *illusion* of a near perfect skin tone. When I discuss the 'art' of applying these three basic products, I am referring to the technique of applying them *without making it obvious to others* that you have applied anything. The effect to strive for is to even out your skin tone – covering or minimizing imperfections – and to create a silky smooth texture on the skin. The most important factor when choosing foundation, concealer and powder is that, once applied, the products look 'invisible' and natural, like 'true skin'. To achieve this effect, it is essential to find the *exact* colours to match your individual skin tone (see page 22 for a discussion of yellow correctors). Some women dislike any form of foundation, either because they experience a 'caked' feel on the skin, or because they fear that wearing foundation will cause blocked pores. Nowadays, however, there are such advanced formulations that you will hardly be aware that you have applied anything to your skin. Carefully select foundation suited to your skin type, and you are sure to be pleased with the result. Many foundation products actually protect the skin from pollutants in the air, and contain sunscreen as well.

Some women apply foundation, but do not use powder to create a silky finish. Many women regard concealer as a product meant only for covering teenage spots or severe blemishes. In order to achieve a truly professional make-up finish, though, *all three* products are necessary. It is essential to realize that make-up will not last on the skin unless it has a properly prepared surface to cling to. Blushers and eye shadows are not formulated to work directly on the skin, or to be applied directly over foundation.

This section explains how to create a base for the application of additional make-up products. Note that your choice of product formulations will determine the order of application, as liquid or creamy products are generally followed by drier ones.

foundation

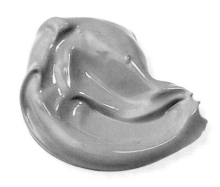

There are two very important aspects to consider when selecting foundation, namely the texture and the colour.

texture

The properties and functions of various foundation formulations (liquids, creams and powders) were discussed on pages 18–19. Experiment with textures from different make-up houses, until you find one you like. Some women like a light, 'barely there' feel on the skin, while others prefer heavier coverage. For some women the most important criteria are that a foundation is quick and easy to apply.

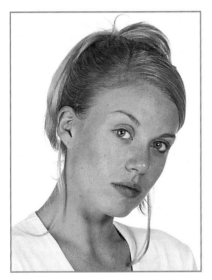

Without foundation unevenness in skin tone and patchiness are visible.

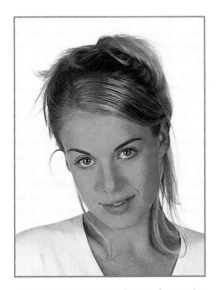

Foundation, concealer and powder create an even skin tone.

colour

This is the single most important factor in choosing foundation. If you fail to find an exact colour match for the base you are creating, you cannot expect any of the additional make-up products to contribute to enhancing the look in the way they should.

Do not leave the colour selection up to the saleslady behind the counter. Be assertive, and insist on checking the colour match carefully yourself. Salesladies are rarely professionally trained make-up artists and are generally geared to selling a particular brand of make-up. Although they may well help you find the closest foundation colour to your skin tone, this is not good enough. What you require is an *exact match*.

The lighting used in department stores also alters colours slightly. A colour that may seem like an exact match inside the store, may be far from ideal once it is seen in natural light. Always, therefore, try to find some natural light in which to check the colour before embarking on an expensive purchase.

Finally, most women go shopping when they have already applied foundation to their skins. In this case, even the most well-intentioned saleslady will find it difficult to identify the true skin tone underneath the foundation. So be brave when going shopping for foundation, and bare your natural skin tone.

The photograph on the left illustrates the application of foundation, concealer and powder matched to the skin tone exactly. Light cover has been applied just to even out the skin tone, and the look is still completely fresh and natural.

testing foundation colour

You may have to test various foundation colours before you find an exact match to your skin. Persevere, however, as a hasty or wrong choice can spoil a look completely. Take a small mirror with you for checking the colour in natural light. Once you have found the correct colour, make a note of the name so that future buys will be simple.

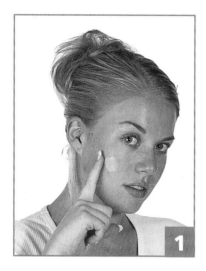

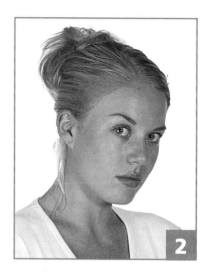

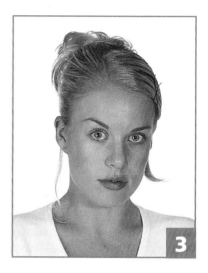

1 Begin your test with a clean skin without any make-up whatsoever, and preferably wait at least 10 minutes after having applied moisturizer. Then dot a small amount of foundation on your fingertip and apply it to your lower cheek area as shown above.

2 Now blend the foundation completely on the cheek. Move to a spot near a window or another source of natural light, and scrutinize the colour of the foundation on your skin in your mirror. Check that the light is evenly distributed across both sides of the face. The correct colour foundation should look next to 'invisible' once applied to the skin.

3 The photograph above shows the right side of the face left bare of foundation, and foundation in the correct colour applied to the left side. Notice how the foundation has not changed the natural skin colour in any way. It has evened out the skin tone quite dramatically, though.

If the colour of the foundation is at all visible, it is incorrect and you will have to start afresh. The photograph on the right demonstrates the wrong colour being used and, although this example has been exaggerated to make a point, you will be amazed at how many women are this careless when selecting foundation.

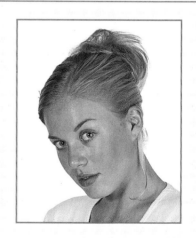

mixing foundation colours

If, when testing, you find a texture that you like, but one colour in the range is too light and the next too dark, consider your own personal mix. Provided you keep to products from the same make-up house, this may very well do the trick. I find that I inevitably have to buy two different

shades, take them home and mix them into a third bottle to obtain my exact colour match. I only mix a certain amount from each bottle into the third, because my skin tends to be paler in winter than in summer, when I spend a little time in the sun.

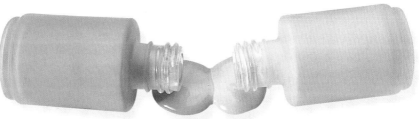

achieving a balance between pink and yellow

A common problem when testing foundation is that a colour may not seem either too pale or too dark, but still does not provide an exact match. In most cases the reason is that the foundation colour is too pink to look like true skin. In fact, the majority of us have skin with yellowy tones, and many commercial foundations simply do not contain enough yellow colouring. You will therefore see many women wearing a pinkish foundation, whilst the skin on their neck and shoulders is clearly yellow-toned. Try to avoid this at all costs, as in these cases foundation looks really artificial.

In the photograph below right, a yellow colour corrector (see page 22) has been added to the foundation to achieve an exact match to the skin tone. Do not be afraid to add yellow, as applying a little too much yellow is still better than walking around with a noticeably pink tint to the face.

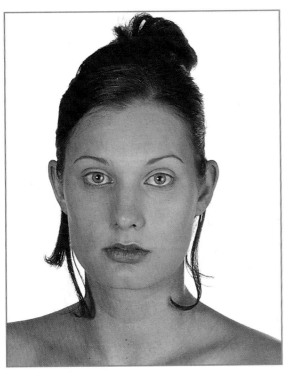

Incorrect – here pink-toned foundation has been applied to yellow-toned skin.

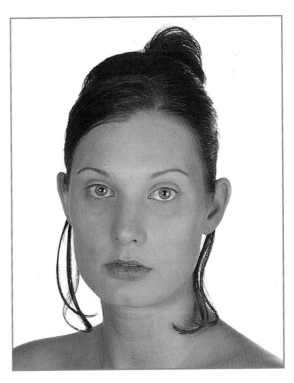

Correct – here yellow-toned foundation has been carefully matched to yellow-toned skin.

applying liquid foundation

It is best to get into the habit of applying moisturizer about 10 minutes before beginning your make-up application. If your skin still feels dry before you start applying foundation, apply a tiny amount of moisturizer to the dry areas. Then use a tissue to blot any excess before proceeding.

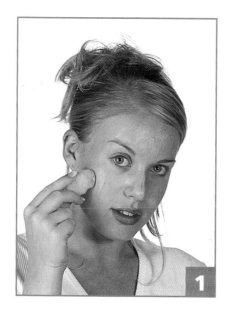

As liquid foundation and liquid concealer are both moist products, the order in which they are applied can vary. I prefer applying foundation first, and then only concealing what the foundation has not already covered. In addition, if concealer is applied first, there is always a chance that some of it will be wiped off as the foundation is blended across the skin.

1 Foundation may be applied using a finger, but for a more even application and a natural finish I recommend using a small, natural sea sponge (see page 9). Wet the sponge first, squeeze out the excess water and then use the damp sponge to spread the foundation evenly across your face. Do not 'dab' foundation on in patches before spreading it, as some foundations dry very quickly, creating an uneven texture.

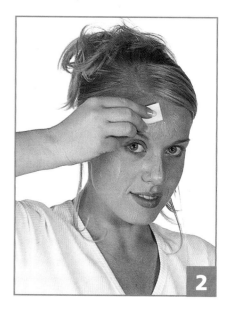

2 After spreading the foundation, use a dry or slightly damp wedge-shaped latex sponge (see page 9) to blend away any fine streaks. Also make sure that the foundation is blended into the indentations around the nose and the eye sockets, and blend carefully just around the edge of the jaw. Eyelids should be covered by foundation, but taking the foundation onto the lips is optional.

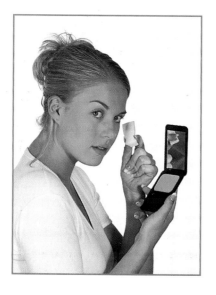

applying powder foundation

If you are using a powder-based foundation formula, you are in fact combining foundation and powder in one product. You will therefore only require concealer in addition to this, and will not need to follow the powdering process outlined on page 43.

Remember that although there are no hard-and-fast rules when it comes to applying make-up, the general rule for the order in which products are used during an application, is to apply moist products first, followed by the drier or powdery products. If you are working with a powder foundation, therefore, you will be applying concealer first (see pages 40–42).

Then, using a latex sponge, gently spread the dry foundation across the entire face. Include the eyelids, exclude the lips and blend the edges just below the jaw.

applying cream foundation

When using a cream-based foundation, concealer may be applied either before or after the foundation. Once again, use a wedge-shaped latex sponge and light strokes to apply the foundation across the face.

Be careful – many women achieve good coverage by using a cream-based foundation, but seldom achieve a finish which looks like true skin. You may feel that you have covered all your flaws and enhanced your look, whereas you may only have created a noticeably heavy and artifical 'mask' which draws attention. Had you not tried to cover everything, and applied lighter coverage, you may have found a much more pleasing natural look. You will be surprised how few people notice the flaws you worry about. Let me repeat that if people notice your make-up before anything else, you have defeated the purpose of wearing it.

for dark skin tones

For dark skins, the principles for testing colour and texture, and for applying foundation remain the same. The colours used will obviously be much darker. If parts of your face are more darkly pigmented than others, you may need to use more than one foundation colour, blending to an even look.

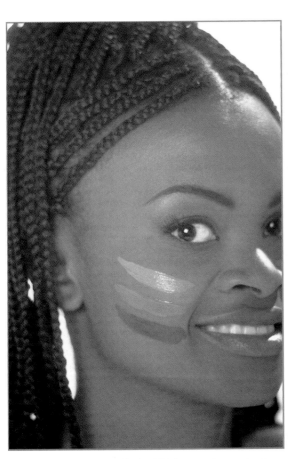

A perfect match on dark skin is very important, as anything even slightly lighter will 'grey' the skin.

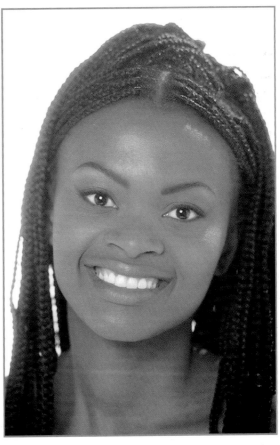

The correct foundation colour evens out the skin tone, whilst retaining a completely natural look.

concealer

Concealer is used on the areas of the face that require more cover than that provided by foundation alone. Applied to eyelids, it also offers a wonderful base for eye shadow, helping it last throughout the day.

choosing concealer

Concealers are available in a various formulations (see page 20). The kind of concealer you choose will depend on what you wish to conceal. For blemishes, a dry stick concealer may be useful, but around the eye area you need a softer product which can be applied without tugging at the skin. Professional make-up artists generally prefer using tubs of cream concealer, which are highly versatile. If you are unable to find this product in a store near you, you may wish to contact a professional supplier (see page 95) to obtain some.

where to apply concealer

A Cover the entire area from the eyelid to the eyebrow

B Mask dark rings under the eyes, staying close to the nose

C Cover any redness still visible through the foundation

D Cover any blemishes

E Avoid applying concealer to this area, as fine lines or wrinkles become emphasized

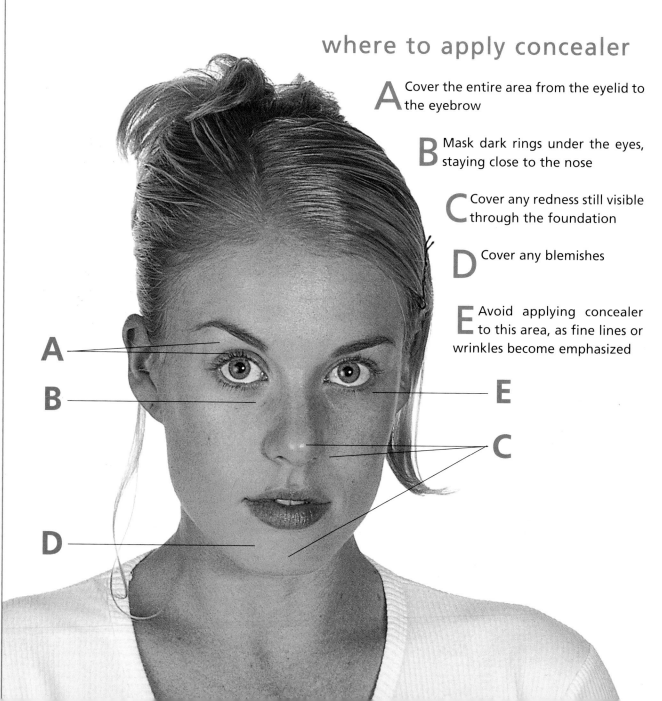

dark rings & eyelids

Every face – even a young one – is given a fresher appearance by applying concealer to the darker skin or 'ring' under the eye, as well as to the eyelids. The skin tone here often seems darker or uneven, owing either to pigmentation or because of the blood in the tiny vessels beneath the skin showing through. To apply concealer, use a soft brush (see page 13) or your finger, if you prefer.

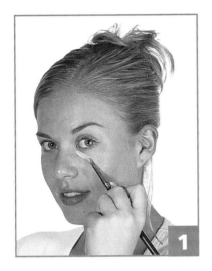 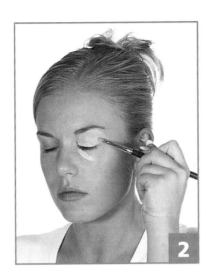 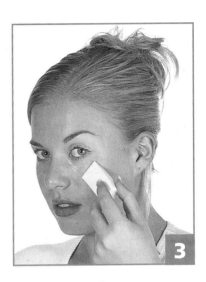

1 Using a small brush, apply concealer below the eyes close to the nose, avoiding the lined area further outwards. The darkest part of the 'ring' is usually at this inner point.

2 Then apply concealer to the entire eyelid as shown above. Extend it all the way up to the eyebrow.

3 To create a neat finish, use a wedge-shaped latex sponge to blend gently.

blemishes

To conceal a blemish or anything prominent, like a mole, for instance, apply concealer to that specific area only by using a small brush.

1 Apply only a tiny dot of concealer, using a small, firm brush made of sable hair.

2 Pat with a fingertip to blend, as a wiping motion is likely to expose whatever you have tried to cover.

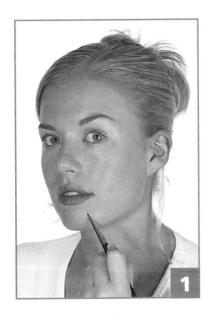 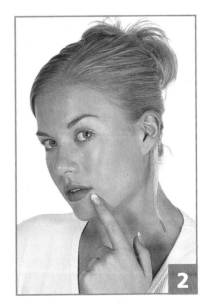

redness

If you are trying to cover a reasonably large patch of skin using concealer, it is of the utmost importance to follow the steps I have outlined below.

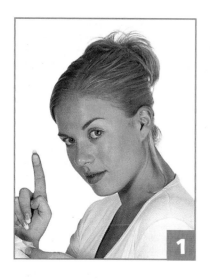
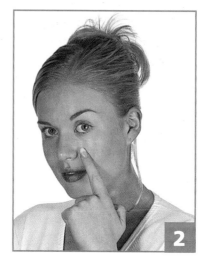

1 Use a light pat to pick up some concealer on your fingertip. Then pat your finger against a tissue to retain only a tiny amount of concealer.

2 Now very gently pat the concealer onto the reddish area, using a motion similar to combining a pat and a wipe.

As so little concealer is applied at a time, no blending should be required. If you have covered an area too heavily, however, use a wedge-shaped sponge to blend lightly.

using concealer on mature skin

Work very carefully when applying concealer to mature skin. A heavy application will not hide lines, but emphasize them instead. Ensure that you choose a soft concealer that blends easily without tugging at the skin. I recommend cream concealers (see page 20).

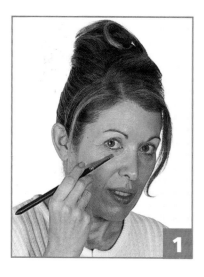
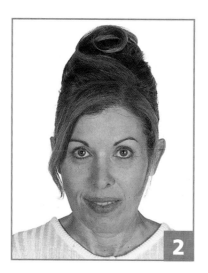
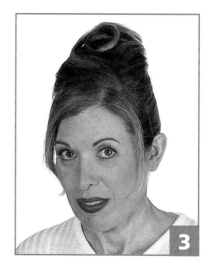

1 Use a small brush, and apply a little concealer below the eyes close to the nose, just avoiding the lined area further outwards.

2 Also apply concealer to the entire eyelid to act as a base for eye shadow. Use a latex wedge to blend gently, creating an even look.

3 The illusion of an even skin tone has been created and a fresher, more youthful look has been achieved.

powder

Applying foundation and concealer can leave the face shiny and a little sticky. The shine can make one look tired, and a sticky surface is not what you need as a base for eye shadow and blusher. Unless you have used a powder-based foundation (see page 19), applying powder is the logical next step. Powder 'sets' the foundation and gives the face a fresh, matte appearance. Not only does it act as a silky base for the application of other products, but it also helps them last. Pressed powder is less messy to carry in your handbag, but does tend to 'build up' on the skin, unlike loose powder. Used with care, it can be useful for quick touch-ups.

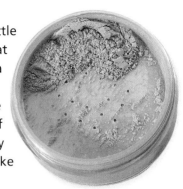

testing powder colour

Although powders are often labelled 'translucent', this does not mean that they are colourless. Aways test powder on your face and check that is does not alter the colour of your foundation. It is a good idea to apply foundation over the entire face, powder only half the face, and then compare the colour. Truly translucent powders are best ordered from professional suppliers (see page 95). Some companies now manufacture a yellow powder (see page 22) that is suitable for use on almost any skin tone, with the exception of very fair skin. This move towards using yellow-toned products is the best way of obtaining a next-to-natural finish.

applying loose powder

Apply a minimal amount of powder to lined areas, and remember to apply powder to the eyelids to create a smooth, silky surface for eye shadow.

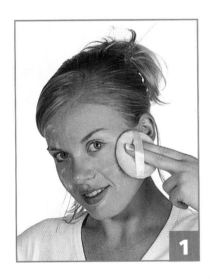

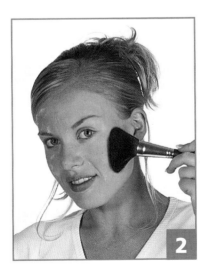

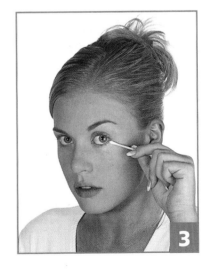

1 Using a good powder puff, apply loose powder in a gentle pressing action to set the foundation.

2 Then use a large, soft powder brush to dust off any excess powder.

3 Using a cotton bud, apply a small amount of powder under the bottom eyelashes. Your eyeliner will blend more easily and last longer.

eyebrows
gain definition

As already discussed on pages 28–33, make-up artists regard eyebrows as a very important facial feature. I discussed and illustrated how to shape eyebrows effectively by removing unwanted hair to create a flattering arch. Refresh your memory, if you like, by referring to this earlier section again, paying special attention to what I termed the 'eye-lift' illusion (see page 28).

In this section I shall be discussing and illustrating make-up application techniques to add definition to eyebrows that have already been shaped correctly by plucking. After applying foundation, concealer and powder to the face (see pages 34–43), the next step is to define the eyebrows.

The order in which the various steps of the make-up application process are followed, is very important. Experiment with a different order if you like, but I think you will find that defining your eyebrows before you proceed to the eyes, cheeks and lips makes a substantial difference in determining the overall 'balance' you aim to create.

Trends in terms of desired eyebrow colour – and even shape – may vary from time to time. There was a time when it was highly fashionable to pluck eyebrows to a very thin line. Some make-up artists working on blonde models bleach the eyebrow hair to achieve very pale, almost invisible brows. In this section I have not attempted to follow specific trends, but rather to set out techniques that are timeless and elegant, and that will suit every woman's face.

If you are not used to applying make-up of any kind to your eyebrows, you may initially feel that your make-up has been 'overdone' or that your eyebrows have been exaggerated too much by the shadow or pencil used to add definition. Always remember, however, that you will be used to seeing your 'old' look when looking in the mirror, and that you are seldom immediately able to objectively judge a 'new' look. Study the faces and the techniques used in this section carefully, and then decide whether you agree that defining eyebrows is important.

Some women may indeed be lucky enough to have thick, full, even eyebrows that require no further defining by make-up. Most of us, however, either have eyebrows that require defining throughout because of sparse, fine hair, or have sparse patches along the length of the brow that require filling in to create an even look.

the importance of defining the eyebrows

Let us begin by seeing what a face looks like without any eyebrows at all (see below left). Do you agree that it looks unbalanced? In the photograph in the centre below, the eyebrows have been included. The eyebrow on the right has been defined, while the eyebrow on the left has been left undefined. Decide for yourself which half of the face looks more balanced and finished.

Even when you opt for a more natural look, with a paler lipstick colour (see below right), the eyebrows still require defining. Again compare the separate halves of the face.

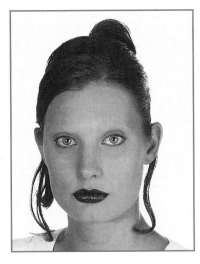

A face without eyebrows looks unbalanced – do you agree?

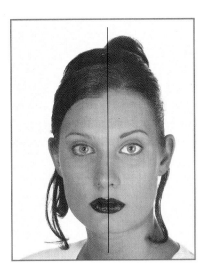

One eyebrow has been defined. Compare the overall balance.

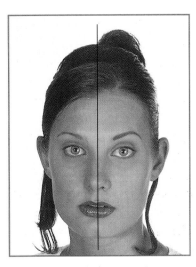

Definition is important, even when creating a more natural look.

choosing colour for your eyebrows

Your present hair colour, whether it be natural, highlighted, coloured, or sun-bleached, will determine the colour you choose for eyebrow make-up.

 Most make-up artists tend to work with black for those with black or dark brown hair.

 Dark brown is used on those with medium to dark brown hair, red hair, or mousy brown to blonde hair.

 Ash-brown is used on those with blonde or very fair hair.

 Rust-brown is only used if the hair is orange-red.

  Charcoal or grey is only used on those with grey hair.

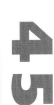

using shadow to define the brows

Unless your eyebrows are very sparse, experiment with using matte, dark eye shadow to define them. In the case of very sparse eyebrows, I recommend using eyebrow pencils (see page 22). In terms of texture, choose eye shadow that does not easily break into dust, or you may risk a rather messy application.

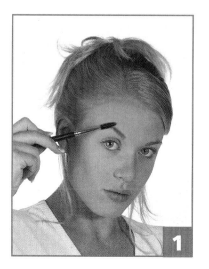 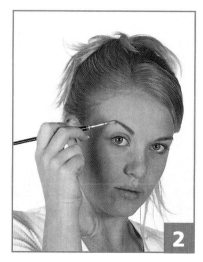 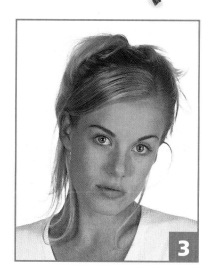

1 First brush the eyebrows into place using a special eyebrow brush or a clean wand-type applicator.

2 Use a small brush of sable hair, or a narrow, angled brush to ensure a neat finish. Lightly dip the brush into the eye shadow. Apply very little powder at a time, dusting off most of the powder you pick up onto a tissue. The real art of defining eyebrows lies in the application of multiple, light, sweeping strokes, thus gradually building up colour to create a natural finish.

3 Working with your natural eyebrow shape and hair growth, aim to achieve a shape which is as close as possible to the ideal. Notice how all the 'gaps' have been filled in and the eyebrow has an even colour throughout.

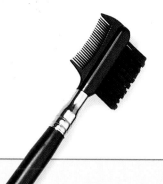

If your eyebrow hair refuses to retain the shape into which you comb it, use a tiny amount of hairspray on your eyebrow brush.

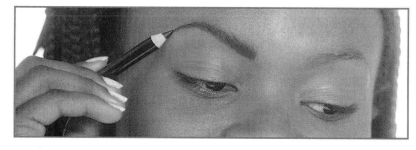

for dark skin tones

Darker skins need a stronger eyebrow than one created by using eye shadow. I recommend using a sharp, hard, dry eyebrow pencil in black. Compare the full-face photograph on page 39 (right).

using eyebrow pencil to define the brows

If you have very little eyebrow hair, applying eye shadow as described on the previous page will look smudgy and unnatural. Rather opt for a good eyebrow pencil (see page 22). If you do not use the correct pencilling technique, though, you may still run the risk of creating an artificial, 'painted' look.

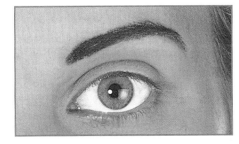

This eyebrow is far too heavily pencilled and looks obviously 'artificial'.

You will be able to create truly natural-looking pencilled eyebrows by:

◆ using proper eyebrow pencils instead of pencil eyeliner
◆ using eyebrow pencils that are hard enough
◆ not applying too much pressure when pencilling
◆ not drawing one solid line.

The correct way to pencil eyebrows is to use a sharp, hard, dry eyebrow pencil and apply the colour in short, light, feathery strokes, forming lots of little hair-like lines on top of each other in the desired eyebrow shape. This does require a certain degree of practice, but once you have mastered the technique, nobody will notice that your brows are not 'real'.

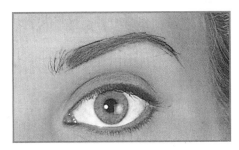

Pencilled correctly, this eyebrow looks elegant yet natural.

using two pencils

To achieve a natural look, you may want to try the technique of combining two pencils of different colours.

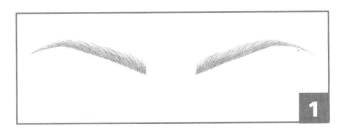

1 First pencil in a series of light, feathery strokes using a brow pencil in a colour matching that of your natural hair.

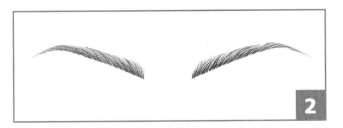

2 Then use a pencil in a slightly darker shade to distribute tiny, darker strokes throughout the length of the eyebrow as illustrated on the left. Concentrate on beginning the strokes along the baseline of the eyebrow throughout the process.

colour
on the face

Whatever your particular colouring in terms of skin tone, eyes, eyebrows and hair, there will always be certain colours that enhance your natural beauty and certain colours that detract from it. Your choice of foundation, concealer and powder, and the importance of matching it to your skin tone has already been discussed on pages 34–43. In this section I shall be discussing and illustrating the use of colour on the face in the form of make-up products like lipsticks, blushers, eyeliners and eye shadows.

For a make-up artist, adding colour to a woman's face is a tricky subject – not because it is difficult to find suitable colour combinations, but because most women grow used to applying certain colours and resist any change that may be suggested. In my experience women invariably dislike colours that they are not accustomed to seeing on their faces.

At this point I would strongly like to encourage you to experiment with different colours on your face. Unless you try out new colours from time to time, you may well become one of the many women who become slaves to the same one or two colours which they use year after year. Not only will your daily make-up application become boring, but you will miss out on the rewards of experimenting with new products and colours which appear on the shelves each season. Although new colour combinations may feel awkward at first, give yourself a chance to get used to them. You may also find that friends begin complimenting you on your looks, not realizing what you have done differently, but simply noticing that you look really good, or fresh and elegant.

'cool' and 'warm' colours

An effective way of determining which make-up colours suit you best, is to separate what we call 'cool' colour palettes from 'warm' colour palettes. Most people will find that one of these colour palettes suits them better than the other – they will either look good in 'cool' tones, or in 'warm' tones. Sometimes the difference can also be very subtle.

telling the difference

Colours that are called 'cool', are given that name because when you look at them, or when you imagine yourself surrounded by them, you experience a 'cool' feeling. So-called 'warm' colours are said to impart a 'warm' feeling. To begin training yourself to be able to look at colours and determine their 'feel' – as being either 'cool' or 'warm' – try using the simple examples given below.

The ocean – a huge mass of blue – is cool, and one can 'feel' its coolness before even touching the water. Blue is thus regarded as a 'cool' colour.

Fire – with flames of orange – is warm, and one can feel the heat without having to go anywhere near the flame. Orange is therefore regarded as a 'warm' colour.

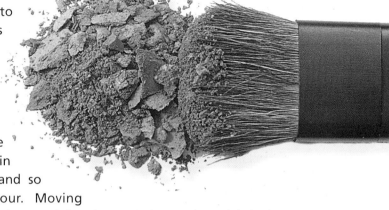

Looking at a wider range of colours, use your imagination to 'feel' either more warmth or more coolness in a colour. Mauve, for example, echoes more of the cool 'ocean' feel than the warm 'fire' feel. Mauve is also closer in colour to blue than it is to orange, and so mauve is regarded as a 'cool' colour. Moving further along the spectrum, one can look at a pink colour. We know that pink is close to mauve, therefore one can say that pink also belongs to the 'cool' group of colours. Yellow, on the other hand, evokes more of the warm 'fire' feel than the cool 'ocean' feel. It is also closer in colour to orange than it is to blue, so yellow can be classified as a 'warm' colour.

When working with make-up, it is a little more complicated to divide colours into 'cool' and 'warm' groups, because instead of looking at simple primary and secondary colours, one uses various make-up 'neutrals' to create illusions on the face. The blusher colours on this page, for example, have been specially selected – the blusher at the top being cool, and the one below being warm. We could simply have chosen pink as cool and orange as warm, but these more 'neutral' blusher colours clearly illustrate the subtle difference between 'cool neutrals' and 'warm neutrals'.

A particular skin tone will either look better combined with cool make-up colours, or with warm make-up colours. If your skin tone is best suited to cool colours, your skin will be referred to as having a blue undertone. On the other hand, if your skin tone is best suited to warm colours, your skin will be referred to as having a yellow undertone.

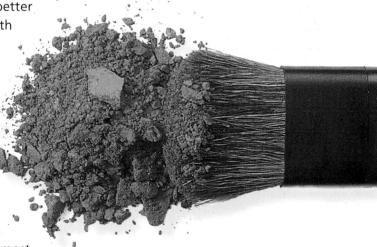

what suits you?

When discussing foundation, concealer and powder on pages 34–43, I spoke of most people as having a yellow surface tone to their skin, and therefore sometimes having to add yellow products to their foundation to achieve a perfect match to their particular skin tone. At this point, however, it is important to clearly distinguish between the 'surface tone' and the 'undertone' of the skin. These two terms refer to different qualities of the skin. Although it may sound contradictory, the majority of us have a yellow surface tone, but a blue undertone.

Clients who consult me professionally often inform me that they have already determined their 'colour type', having, for instance, analyzed the colour of the skin on the inside of their forearms. Quite often, however, they have made an inaccurate assessment, because they have been looking at the yellow of their skin's surface tone instead of the skin's particular undertone.

To help solve this problem, I suggest that you use pages 52 and 53 in this book, as well as two rather bright lipstick colours (see below right) to conduct a very practical test.

doing 'the colour test'

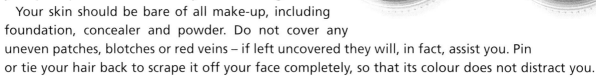

When you conduct this test, make sure that your face is evenly lit by natural light. Try standing near a window, but not in bright or direct sunlight. Use a mirror large enough for you to see your whole face, including the neck and shoulders. Bare your shoulders, as a coloured garment may influence your perception of the colours you are testing.

Your skin should be bare of all make-up, including foundation, concealer and powder. Do not cover any uneven patches, blotches or red veins – if left uncovered they will, in fact, assist you. Pin or tie your hair back to scrape it off your face completely, so that its colour does not distract you.

If you do not trust your own judgement, try doing this test in the company of a couple of good friends who will be honest and objective. Be careful when selecting someone to help you, though, as they may subconsciously choose the colour they prefer, and not the colour that suits you best.

To do the test, you will compare orange and pink. It is essential that the colours used are of a similar intensity, though, or your judgement will be inaccurate. You will need an orange and a pink lipstick similar to those shown above, as well as pages 52 and 53 of this book.

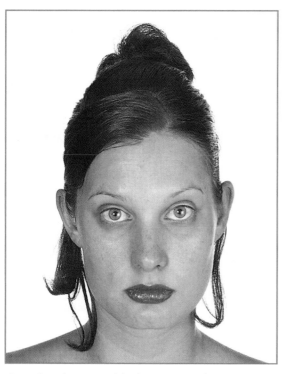

A cool undertone with the wrong *colour.*

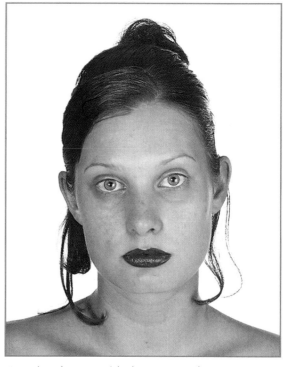

A cool undertone with the correct *colour.*

step-by-step

1 Turn the book and hold it so that the pink page (page 52) is below your chin, and the orange page (page 53) is hanging down towards the floor. Look at your face in the mirror with only the pink page next to it, paying attention to your face, not to the page of colour. See how the pink colour interacts with any imperfections like unevenness in skin tone, blotches, blemishes or red veins. Do these imperfections show up more, or do they seem to fade?

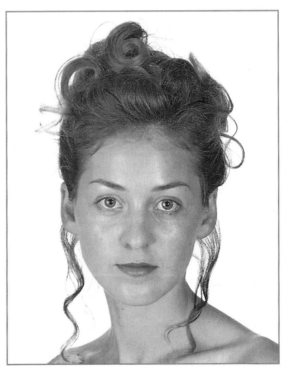

2 Now follow the same procedure again – this time holding the orange page (page 53) below your chin, with the pink page (page 52) hanging out of sight. Look at how the orange colour interacts with your skin, and with any imperfections.

3 For this step and the next, you will require lipstick. Firstly, apply the pink lipstick, and again hold the pink page next to your face. Study the effect the colour has on your appearance.

4 Use a good make-up remover to remove all traces of the pink lipstick from your lips. Then apply the orange lipstick, and hold the orange page next to your face.

The *wrong* colour will make the skin around blemishes appear paler, and make the blemishes seem more noticeable. Your skin may also look blotchy, especially around the mouth area.

The *correct* colour seems to give the skin a radiant glow and it creates a generally harmonious look, with blemishes becoming less noticeable.

The photographs on this page and the previous page illustrate the effect achieved by applying either the wrong or the correct colour to the face.

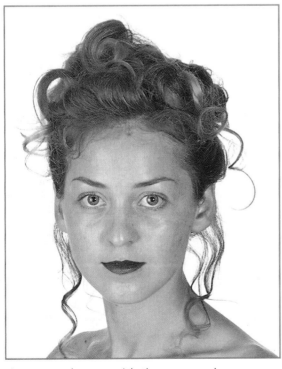

A warm undertone with the wrong *colour.*

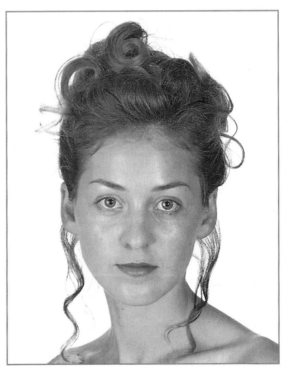

A warm undertone with the correct *colour.*

cool & warm 'neutrals'

It is quite easy to classify bright, clear pink and orange, like the lipsticks in tubs used on page 50, as either 'cool' or 'warm'. Page 52 of this book is also clearly 'cool', whilst page 53 is clearly 'warm'.

When it comes to making the distinction in terms of make-up colours, however, things are not that simple. To create a natural, elegant, timeless look, make-up artists do not use bright blues, greens, pinks, oranges or yellows, as these colours are too bright to create any feeling of depth on the face. To create illusion around the eyes, as well as on the cheeks and lips, make-up artists need to shade or darken certain areas to make them recede, and highlight other areas to make them seem more prominent. To do this most successfully, 'neutral' colours are used, especially on the eyes and cheeks.

Gaining an understanding of the term 'neutral' colour is therefore essential – as is being able to see the difference between a 'cool neutral' colour and a 'warm neutral' colour. Looking at a range of neutral colours, like different shades of brown, for example, and dividing them into cool and warm shades can be quite tricky. To simplify the process, I suggest asking yourself what I call 'the colour question': *Can I see more pink and mauve tones in this colour, or more orange and yellow tones?*

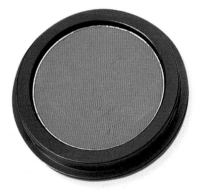

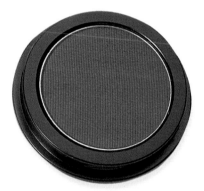

a *Pink and mauve are cool colours. This brown has subtle mauve tones, and so it belongs in a cool palette.*

b *Orange and yellow are warm colours. This brown has subtle orange tones, and so it belongs in a warm palette.*

The same 'colour question' can be asked of these five lipstick colours.

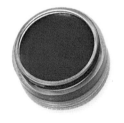
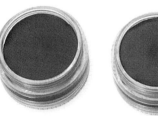
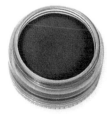

cool reds

*primary red
(not influenced by
cool or warm tones
and can be worn
by everyone)*

warm reds

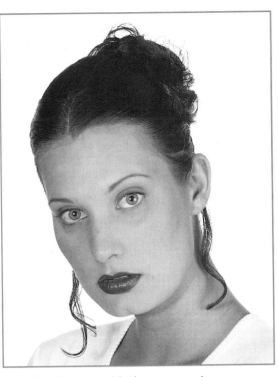

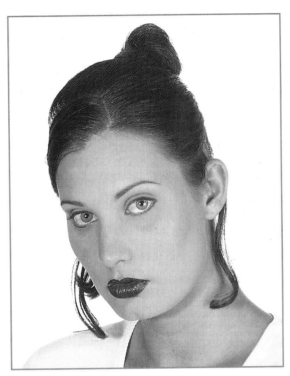

A cool undertone with the wrong *colours.*

A cool undertone with the correct *colours.*

Although certain colours may be your favourites, because you know they look good and you have become used to them, be brave enough to experiment. Once you have identified whether warm or cool colours suit you best, try some variations within the warm or cool palette. You may discover that colours you never thought of using look great on you. On the following two pages I have set out the various make-up colours I recommend in terms of warm and cool palettes.

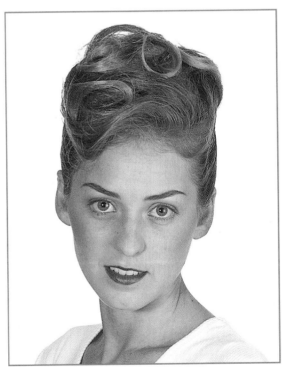

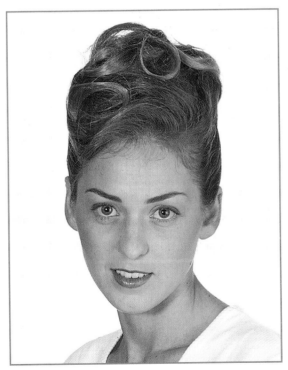

A warm undertone with the wrong *colours.*

A warm undertone with the correct *colours.*

cool

eye shadow

lipstick

blusher

silver

grey

cool make-up colours

If you have completed 'the colour test' (see pages 50–51) and determined that your skin has a *cool* undertone, select your make-up colours from the palette set out on this page. Note that there are three categories of colours: one for eye shadows, one for lipsticks, and one for blushers. You could even consider taking these charts with you as a guide when shopping for make-up.

warm

eye shadow   lipstick   blusher

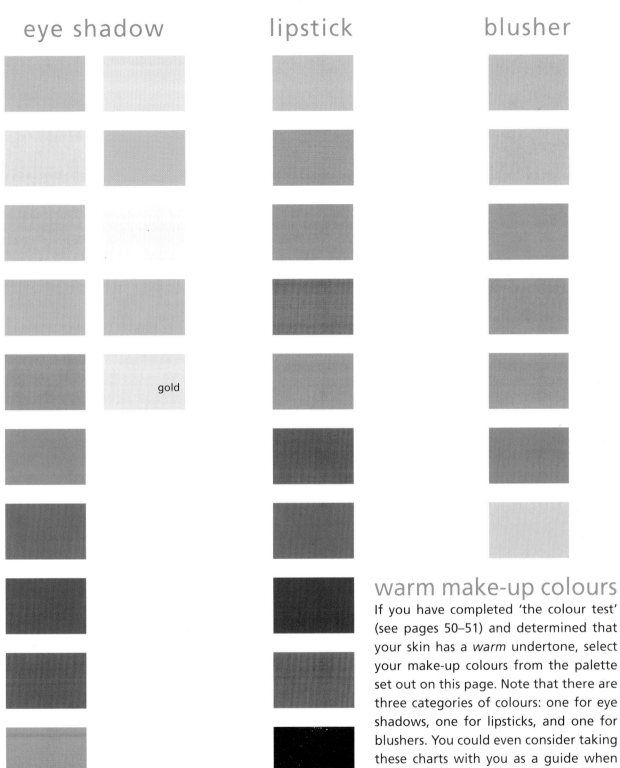

gold

warm make-up colours

If you have completed 'the colour test' (see pages 50–51) and determined that your skin has a *warm* undertone, select your make-up colours from the palette set out on this page. Note that there are three categories of colours: one for eye shadows, one for lipsticks, and one for blushers. You could even consider taking these charts with you as a guide when shopping for make-up.

eyes
do the talking

A woman's eyes are her most expressive facial feature. When we communicate, we look into each others' eyes. And eyes can be used most effectively to convey a wide range of emotions, depending on the setting – from the ballroom to the boardroom. Learning how eye make-up techniques can influence the image you project is thus very important. Keep your 'evening eyes' for glamorous occasions, and look professional, yet natural and elegant at work.

Eye make-up should be used to enhance your eyes – in terms of their colour and shape – and not to provide 'decoration'. If your eye shadow attracts more attention than your eyes themselves, the purpose of the application has been defeated. Matte, neutral shades applied in the right places will draw someone's gaze into the eyes themselves. Shimmery pale blue shadow from eyelid to eyebrow will only draw attention to itself.

Applying eye make-up is probably the trickiest of all the techniques to be mastered. Practise this part of your make-up application and learn what works for you.

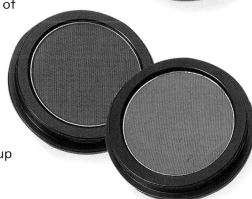

the art of illusion

The key to the art of eye make-up application is being able to successfully create illusions. Any 'faults' you perceive – although other people may not regard them as such – can be minimized, and the illusion of more beautiful and youthful, bright, expressive eyes can be created. No matter whether you feel your eyes are 'too small', 'too round' or 'too deep-set' or whether you have 'too little' or 'too much' eyelid, or close-set or wide-set eyes – each of these factors will be discussed.

highlighting and shading

The two basic techniques used to enhance the eye's natural shape are *highlighting* and *shading*. Without question the most effective colours to combine with this technique are matte, neutral shades, such as those at the top of this page, namely white or cream highlighter, and a warm or cool shading colour, such as those shown above. Always bear in mind this basic rule: *light brings an area forward and makes it appear larger or more prominent, while dark makes an area recede, or makes it appear smaller and less prominent.* To create the desired illusion, it is essential to work with light and dark together.

eye-shadow colours

cool   **warm**

highlighters
(use any of the three pale colours below, or any other light colours from the cool palette)

highlighters
(use any of the three pale colours below, or any other light colours from the warm palette)

shading colours   ## shading colours

Your choice of colours for highlighting and shading is not determined by the colour of your eyes, but by determining whether your skin has a cool or warm undertone. If you have not already identified the colour of your skin undertone, do so now before continuing. The technique used to do this is set out on pages 50–51.

Blue eye shadow is most certainly not the best way of enhancing blue eyes, nor green eye shadow the best for green eyes. In fact, blue and green eye shadows are usually highly problematic, and should be used with great discretion. In this book, for instance, I have used blue only to line eyes (see page 48), and green to create a fun, funky evening look for a young girl (see page 87).

Once you have determined whether you have a cool or warm skin undertone, use the charts of cool and warm colours supplied on this page to help you select effective colours to be used for highlighting and shading. You will note that most of these colours are matte, neutral shades, but that they still offer you a wide range of choices.

Please note, also, that these are not the *only* colours I recommend – they are merely offered as a guide within the cool and warm ranges. If your favourite colour does not appear here, do not despair!

key

▼ not recommended for deep-set or small eyes
● preferably for younger skin or evening application only

copper

grey   silver   gold

eyelid shape

Before deciding which part of the eye area to highlight and which part to shade, it is essential to examine the shape of your eyes and eyelids. Everyone can begin by applying highlighter to the browbone just below the eyebrow, but when it comes to the eyelid, one is faced with a choice. Depending on the amount of visible eyelid, you will decide whether to highlight or shade your lid. Do you want the lid to look more prominent, or less prominent? Study your eyes in a mirror and compare their shape to the illustrations below. Look straight ahead, and do not lift or drop your chin. Which illustration most closely resembles your eye, especially in terms of the shape of the lid?

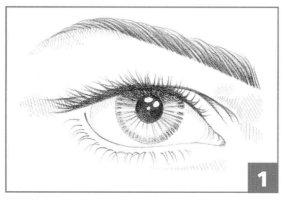

Little or no eyelid is visible.

1 If your eyes most closely resemble illustration 1 in shape, with little or no visible eyelid, you will want to create the illusion of there being more eyelid. You should therefore be applying highlighter on the lid to bring it forward and make it more prominent. You will shade only the crease of the eye, taking the shading colour outwards to join the outside corner of the eye.

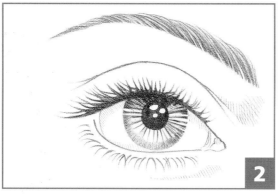

The eyelid is too prominent or puffy, or too much of it protrudes.

2 If your eyes most closely resemble illustration 2 in shape, you will want to create the illusion of there being less visible eyelid, or of it being less protruding or puffy. You should therefore be shading the lid as well as the crease of the eye. In this case, highlighter will only be applied below the eyebrow, and not on the eyelid itself.

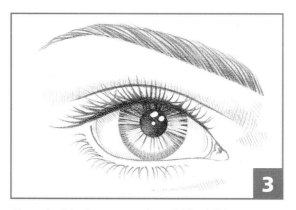

Here the ideal amount of eyelid is visible.

3 If your eyes most closely resemble illustration 3 in shape, you are lucky to have the choice of either highlighting or shading the lid area. You will still be shading the crease of the eye, and applying highlighter under the eyebrow.

using shadow to create shape

On the previous page you will have learnt how to determine whether your eyelids should be highlighted or shaded, or whether you are free to choose either highlighting or shading. I have not yet discussed the *shape* in which highlighter and shading colour should be applied, however.

To determine the shape of the shading, you need to study not the shape of the eye as before, but *the shape of the surrounding skin and bone structure.*

Study the four illustrations below, and look at the differences and the similarities between them. In illustrations a and b, the eyelids have been highlighted. In illustrations c and d, the eyelids have been shaded. Using what you have learnt about the shape of your own eyelids on the previous page, you will study either illustrations a and b, or illustrations c and d.

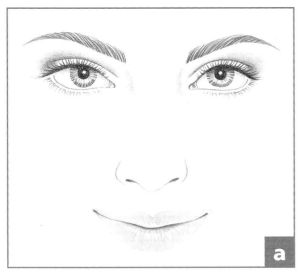

The lid is highlighted, and the crease is shaded. The shading follows the rounded crease of the lid and then comes down to the outer corner of the eye.

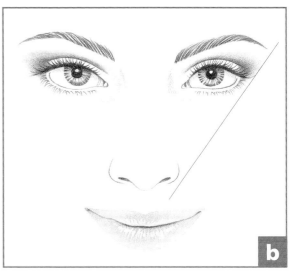

The lid is highlighted, and the crease is shaded. The shading colour extends upwards and outwards into a 'wing' shape in line with the end of the brow.

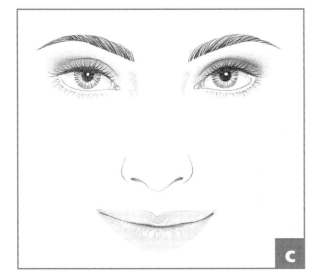

The eyelid and the crease are both shaded. The shading follows the rounded crease of the lid and then comes down to the outer corner of the eye.

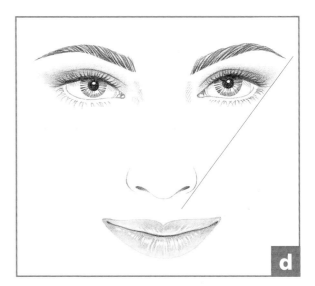

The eyelid and the crease are both shaded. The shading colour extends upwards and outwards into a 'wing' shape in line with the end of the brow.

choosing a suitable shape

The best way of finding out which of the two shapes suits you personally, is to apply the 'rounded' shading shape (either a or c on the previous page) to one eye, and the 'winged' shading shape (either b or d) to the other eye. Then compare your eyes, and decide which shape is most enhancing. You may find that you are lucky enough to be able to use either shape, and are not limited to one shape alone (i.e. you may be able to use both a and b, OR c and d, OR any of the four).

The rounded application technique (either a or c) suits most people, unless you have very little space between the crease of your eye and your eyebrow. In this case, you only have room to work outwards, so use the winged shape.

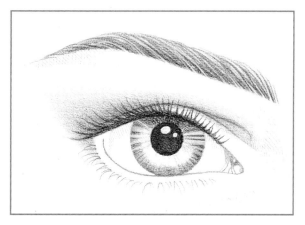

Use the winged application technique with care. It is best used on younger eyes, or where the skin towards the outside of the eye is firm and does not sag at all.

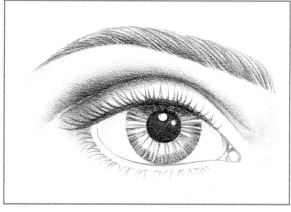

If your browbone prominently curves around the eye as illustrated above, avoid applying shadow in a winged shape.

If you have applied too much eye shadow and the colour has gone darker than you would have liked, do not rub at the colour to tone it down. Rather dip a ball of cotton wool in your loose powder and gently blend until the colour has lightened. Once you have achieved the desired shade, dust off excess loose powder.

Left: Cotton buds are very useful for neatening the edges of your eye-shadow shape, especially if you are applying shadow in the the winged shape extending outwards.

wide-set eyes and close-set eyes

If you have particularly wide-set or close-set eyes, you may want to further refine your application technique. To avoid confusion, all the illustrations below show the eyelid having been highlighted. If your eyelid is better suited to being shaded (see page 61), replace the highlighter with a shading colour. Also retain the rounded or winged shape as appropriate (see pages 61–62).

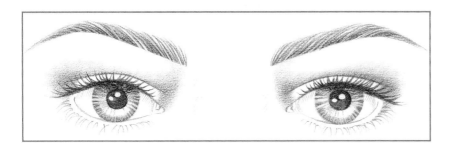

For wide-set eyes suited to the rounded application shape, extend the colour inwards from the crease and up towards the eyebrow to create the illusion of less space between the eyes.

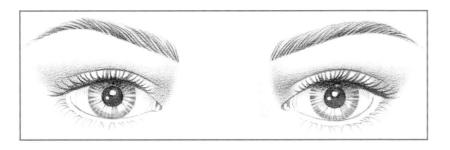

For wide-set eyes suited to the winged application shape, extend the shading colour inwards from the crease and up towards the eyebrow to create the illusion of less space between the eyes.

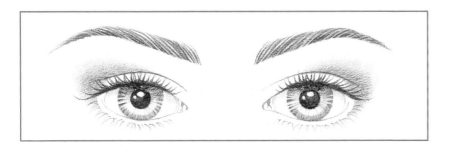

For close-set eyes suited to the rounded application shape, avoid shading the inner part of the eye crease and ensure that the shading begins and fades gently – not along hard lines.

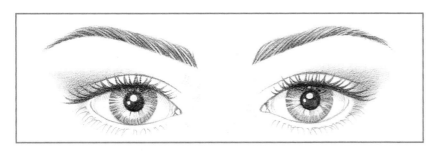

For close-set eyes suited to the winged application shape, avoid shading the inner part of the eye crease and ensure that the shading begins and fades gently – not along hard lines.

For eyes that are deep-set or small, avoid using dark shading colours (marked with a ▼ on the colour chart on page 59), as these will accentuate the 'flaws'. Keep your eyes lighter – even for evenings – and darken your blusher and lipstick.

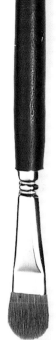

using brushes to apply eye shadow

When using brushes to apply powder eye shadow, use a dome-shaped brush to apply the powder, and a flat-topped brush to blend hard 'edges' or 'bands' of colour. If there is not much space between the eye and the eyebrow, use a smaller brush to ease application.

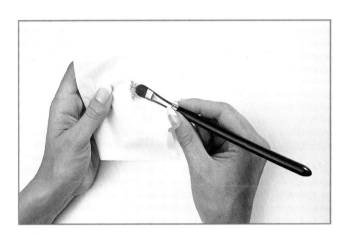

Hold the dome-shaped brush on its side as shown on the left, and gently sweep it across the shadow. This will allow the powder to be picked up evenly along the graduated shape, as it clings to the individual hairs. When the brush is swept across the skin, the powder will be spread out evenly, and not deposited only in one patch.

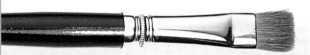

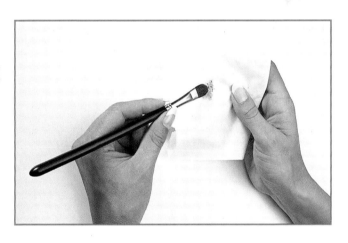

Always dust the excess shadow from the brush onto a tissue before bringing the brush up to your eye. If you have done this, there will be no excess powder to fall messily below the eye.

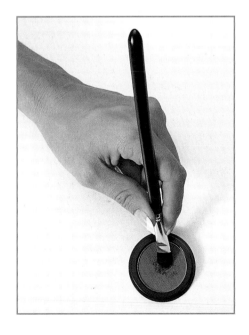

Do not 'dip' your brush into the eye shadow from the top as shown (left), as the powder will then only be picked up by the brush tip. The angle at which the brush hits the product here also causes the compacted powder to break up into small pieces. Much of the product will be wasted, and it will become increasingly difficult and messy to work with.

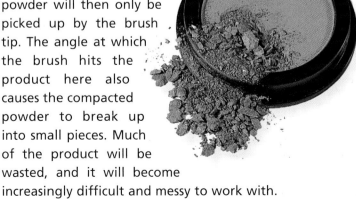

applying eye shadow

Remember that any eye shadow product requires a base on the skin to cling to. If you have not already done so, gently apply and blend concealer over the entire eyelid (see pages 41 and 42), and then powder well (see page 43). Make sure that the lid feels powdery and silky – not tacky – before beginning an eye-shadow application.

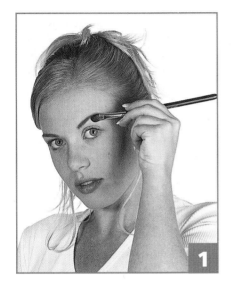

1 Using a medium to large dome-shaped brush, apply your chosen highlighter below the eyebrow.

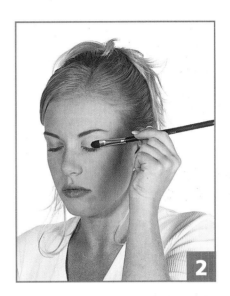

2 Depending on the shape of your eyelid (see page 60), also apply highlighter to the lid across the bulge of the eye and all the way down to the lashes. If you will be shading your eyelid instead of highlighting it, move on to the next stage.

Use a smaller dome-shaped brush to apply the colour you have chosen for shading. When applying darker colours, a smaller brush is easier to work with.

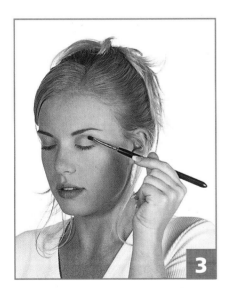

3 Using the technique described on page 61, sweep the brush along the crease of the eyelid in the curve as shown. Apply the shadow keeping the brush flat against the skin and using the entire length of the hair, not only the tip of the brush. Work the colour along the eye crease evenly. If you are shading your lid rather than highlighting it (see page 61), now also work the shadow across your eyelid all the way down to the lashes.

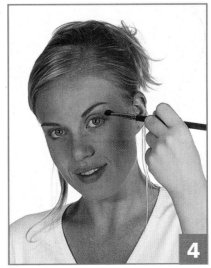

4 Now use a flat-topped brush for blending. Gently sweep across the areas where the light and dark colours meet, to blend and soften the edges as well as to even out the distribution of the eye shadow.

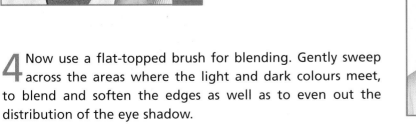

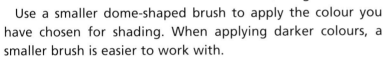

the importance of blending

To illustrate the importance of blending eye shadow colours after application, I have here included two photographs in which I use a combination of brown and black as shading colours.

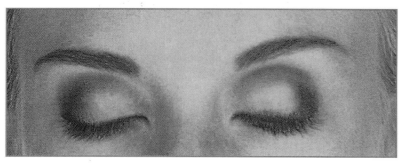

On the eyelid on the left the colours have been blended and the 'hard edges' have been softened. This is the effect to be aimed for.

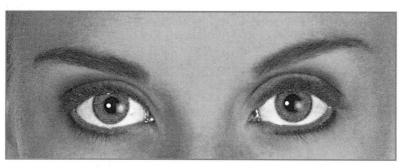

When the eyes are open, the softening effect of blending is clear. Compare the softened line below the eye on the left to the hard line on the right.

Look at the eye on the right in the top photograph. You will notice that highlighter has been applied to the brow-bone, as well as to the eyelid. The prominence of the eyelid is therefore being enhanced.

Brown eye shadow has been applied to the crease of the eye in a rounded shape, and the brown colour has been brought down in a curve to the outer corner of the eye.

Black eye shadow has been applied to the outer corner of the eyelid only, in a slightly curved shape. Note how the eye shadow does not extend beyond the outer corner. The black and brown shadows have not yet been blended on the right side, so that you are still able to distinguish the two separate colours.

using shimmer

Eye shadows containing a shimmer or pearly finish should be used with great care. For example, if a shimmer colour is applied to a puffy or wrinkled area on the eye, sparkle in the colour will illuminate the puffiness or wrinkle and make it more obvious, even though the base colour of the shimmer may be dark. Here the shimmer finish can defeat the purpose of applying dark shading, because it can draw attention to the exact area you wish to make less prominent. For mature skin, I strongly recommend keeping to matte neutrals only, to create as youthful an illusion as possible. Even on younger skins, I generally use shimmer eye shadows only for evening make-up, where lighting is less harsh than daylight, unless I am working for a magazine requiring a specific look. Using shimmer for fun, funky evening looks is discussed on pages 86–87.

using colour

As discussed and illustrated on the previous pages, I strongly recommend keeping to neutral colours like warm or cool browns to create effective illusions, yet natural-looking eye make-up. There are times, however, when some colour may be appropriate to add a little glamour. Use your discretion, though, as you do not want your eye make-up drawing more attention than your eyes.

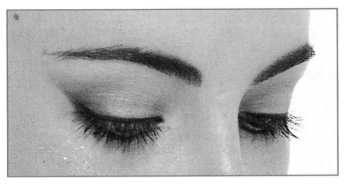

To create these funky 'evening eyes', deep purple eyeliner is used, and the colour is echoed in the extended 'wing' shape.

Evening make-up offers the best opportunity for adding colour to the eyes. In dim lighting in a restaurant or theatre, for example, the face can sometimes look rather pale and 'washed out'. Now is the time to use eye shadow in a brighter colour to frame the eyes – close to the lashes – in the same way in which you would use eyeliner. Dark blue, dark purple or dark green can be highly effective, and you will notice that I have included these colours in the colour charts for eyeliner on page 68.

'evening eyes'

The only difference between make-up techniques used to create daytime and evening looks, is that darker shading colours can be used at night. The application technique remains exactly the same. Compare the two photographs below, where a very glamorous evening look has been created using black eye shadow applied in a rounded shape.

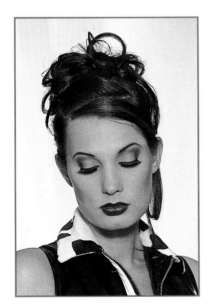

Black shadow and false eyelashes create a dramatic look.

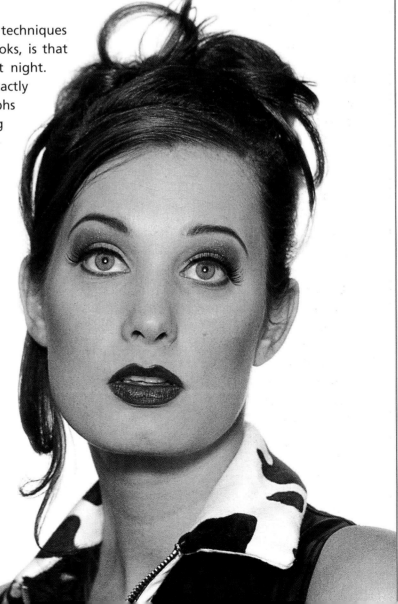

eyeliner

The function of eyeliner is to frame and define the eyes, drawing attention to them. Note clearly that I say attention should be drawn to the eyes – not to the eye make-up. Never apply such harsh eyeliner that it draws attention to itself, rather than to the eye it is enhancing.

To line eyes subtly yet effectively, many make-up artists prefer using eye shadow instead of eye pencil. Pencils used for lining eyes should be soft and smudgy (see page 23), so that they do not drag at the delicate skin around the eye. This does mean that eyeliner pencils contain a fair amount of oil, though, which melts with heat.

A line of eye shadow is softer and easier to blend than pencil. During application there is no tugging at the skin, and shadow does not melt or smudge in humid climates as often as pencil does.

choosing eyeliner colours

Colours used to line eyes should always be subtle and, once again, the colours are determined by your natural skin tone and hair colour. In certain cases, brighter colours may be applied, but this should not become a habit, and colour should be used with great care. The chart given here indicates the range of eyeliner colours I recommend.

 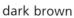 dark brown

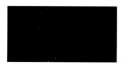 black

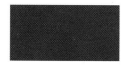 charcoal

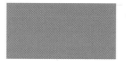 navy/dark blue*

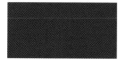 teal*

 dark green*

 purple*

- ◆ for fair to medium brown hair, use dark brown eyeliner
- ◆ for medium to dark brown hair, use black or dark brown eyeliner
- ◆ for red hair, use black or dark brown eyeliner
- ◆ for black hair, use black eyeliner
- ◆ for grey hair or cool skin tones, use charcoal eyeliner
- ◆ for a more colourful look, or for evenings*, use navy/dark blue, teal, dark green or purple

For evening glamour, one sometimes wants to use a little colour around the eyes (see opposite). As a variation, first use a dark framing colour, such as black or dark brown to define the eyes with a very fine line. Then blend a lighter colour, such as blue or green over and just outside this very dark line. The colours should overlap slightly.

using eye shadow as eyeliner

When you are using eye shadow to frame the eyes, I recommend that you use a high-quality compacted powder formulation that does not break up into dust as you apply it. The dustiness is messy, and could irritate the eyes. Some make-up artists prefer working with a wet brush, but I like working with the dry shadow to ensure a soft, smoky edge and no hard lines. A small brush made of sable hair is the ideal applicator (see page 12).

applying eyeliner with a brush

The following steps will show you how and where to apply eyeliner.

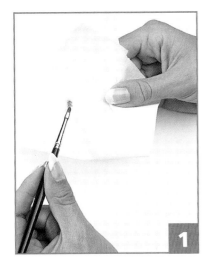

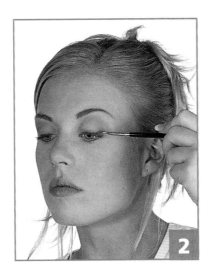

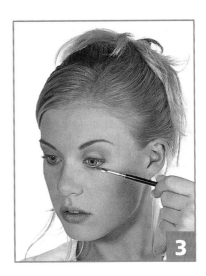

1 Always dust excess powder from the brush onto a tissue to leave very little powder on the brush.

2 Apply a line of shadow to the top lid, getting as close to the lashes as possible.

3 Apply a soft line of eye shadow under the eye, joining the top line at the outside corner.

4 Use a clean cotton bud to soften any hard lines you have created.

using colour to line eyes

If you want to add some colour to your eyes on occasion, eyeliner offers the perfect opportunity. By using colour only in your eyeliner, and not in your eye shadow, you can still create illusion whilst not drawing attention away from the eyes themselves. Suitable lively colours for use as eyeliner have been included in the colour chart (see opposite). An example of blue eyeliner used to pick up the colour of clothing and to enhance the colour of the eye can also be seen in the photograph on page 48.

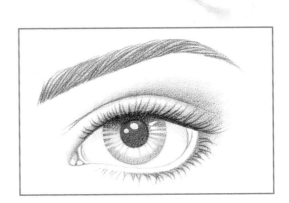

Eyeliner offers the best opportunity of adding colour to an otherwise neutral palette.

eyeliner variations

Eyeliner applied all the way round the eye does not suit everyone. The size and shape of the eye will determine the most effective way of framing.

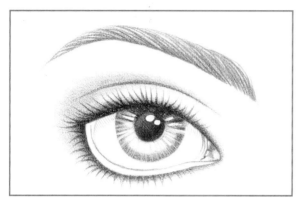

A large eye can be framed all the way round the top and bottom, using black or a dark framing colour.

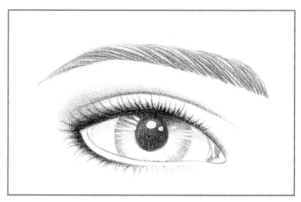

Medium and small eyes can seem smaller if they are framed all the way round. Frame the top, but only the outer section of the lower lid, if at all.

pencil eyeliner

Make sure that your eyeliner pencil has a soft and creamy consistency (see page 23), so that you are able to blend the line without stretching the skin around the eye too much. If you have just sharpened your pencil, use a tissue to round off any sharp edges. This will limit the danger of scratching the skin, and a rounded tip will give a more natural finish.

If your lashes are sparse, avoid using pencil eyeliner, as the line created will appear thick and unnatural.

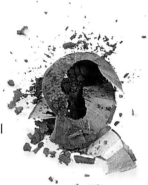

liquid eyeliner

This only looks effective if you are able to create a clean, thin line. Liquid eyeliner does not suit everyone, or every occasion – ask an honest friend for her opinion. If you do decide to use this liquid, make sure that you practise the application until you have perfected the technique. In addition, obtain a high-quality liquid eyeliner brush instead of the usual applicator supplied with the product. Rest your elbow on a working surface to steady your hand.

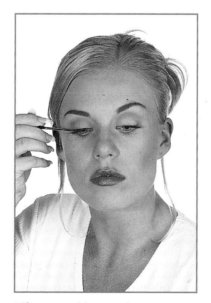

Lift your chin so that you are looking down into a mirror.

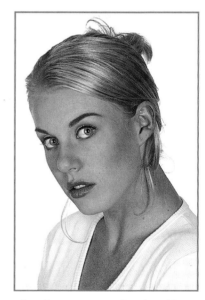

The line you apply should be thinner where it begins and ends.

mascara

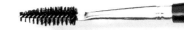

Mascara darkens and thickens the eyelashes, and makes them appear longer. Many make-up artists, myself included, only apply mascara to the top lashes for everyday make-up applications. Mascara applied to the lower lashes often smudges under the eye, and looks messy halfway through the day. The lower lashes can also create a shadow under the eye, which is accentuated by applying mascara to them. If you already have darkish rings under your eyes, this will draw attention to them. Experiment with leaving the lower lashes bare. If this feels strange and your lower lashes are very fair, it may be better to have them tinted by a beauty therapist, rather than applying mascara to them.

choosing mascara colour

Though brightly coloured eyelashes become a fashion trend from time to time (see page 87), I recommend keeping to dark brown or black mascara for everyday wear.

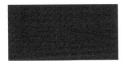 dark brown

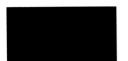 black

 charcoal

- ◆ for fair hair, use dark brown mascara
- ◆ for red hair, use dark brown or black mascara
- ◆ for mousy brown to black hair, use black mascara
- ◆ for grey hair, use charcoal or black mascara

> If you are using lash thickener, allow it to dry before applying mascara over it.

applying mascara

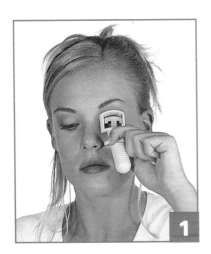

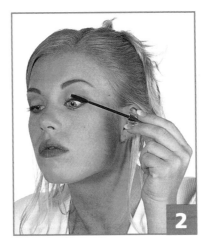

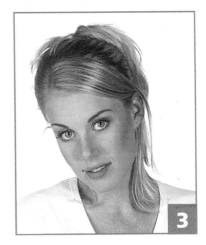

1 If you are using an eyelash curler, first curl the lashes, holding them in the curled position for 10–20 seconds.

2 Lifting your chin while looking down, stroke the mascara through your top lashes, combing them upwards.

3 To achieve a neat finish and reach the base of the lashes, use your free hand to lift the outer corner of the lid.

cheeks
get the blush

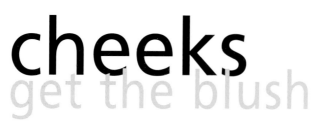

Applying make-up to her cheeks can present a woman with several tricky decisions. First and foremost, you need to decide *why* you are applying blusher to your face. Are you trying to enhance the shape of your face by contouring and creating illusions, or are you merely attempting to add some healthy-looking colour because you feel you look too pale? Both of these are valid reasons for applying blusher to your face, but they call for different choices of colour and different application techniques.

In terms of enhancing the shape of your face, blusher can be used in several ways. It can be applied in places where it serves to give more definition and prominence to cheekbones, for instance. Conversely, blusher can be used to shade and darken, or visually 'soften' cheekbones that may already be felt to be too prominent. It may also be used to create the illusion of contours that 'slim' an otherwise roundish face.

In terms of adding colour to the face, the positioning of blusher often clearly separates the amateurs from the professionals. If adding colour is your main reason for applying blusher to your cheeks, pay particular attention to the discussion on page 76.

As blusher can fulfil these two separate functions – that of contouring, and that of adding colour – one can, in fact, divide the application process into two separate stages. If your cheeks already possess natural colour, you may not need to add blusher colour to achieve a healthy-looking glow. On the other hand, if your cheekbones are already quite sharply defined, you may not need to add any form of contouring, only a little colour.

It is important, therefore, to study the shape of your face and decide *why* you are applying blusher. Then use this section to guide you in terms of *where* to apply it, and *which colours* to choose to create the particular effect you desire. In my experience most women find that they can define or contour, as well as adding colour. The first stage of the application will thus consist of using neutral colours to define the shape of your face. The second stage will involve adding colour.

Whatever your particular reason for applying blusher to your cheeks, the *art* lies in being able to position the colour in the exact area to create the desired effect, without making the blusher colour 'stripy' or obvious in any way.

blusher colours

cool

highlighters

warm

highlighters

shading colours

shading colours

choosing blusher colours

As you did when selecting eye-shadow colours, you will need to choose blusher colours from either the warm or cool palette, depending on the undertone of your skin. If you have not yet identified your undertone colour, you will need to do so now before continuing (see pages 48–55).

When faced with a blusher colour, ask yourself the following question: *can I see more pink or mauve tones in this blusher, or can I see more orange and yellow tones?* Pink and mauve tones suggest a cool colour and orange and yellow tones suggest a warm colour. If you have a cool skin undertone, select blusher from the cool colour palette. If you have a warm skin undertone, select blusher from the warm colour palette.

key

■ preferably for evening applications – not suitable for fair skin tones

❱ to add natural colour to the face after shading colours have been applied

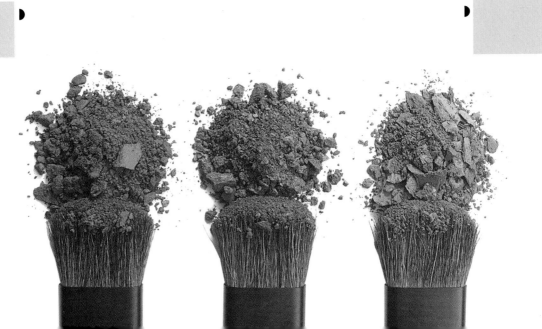

highlighting and shading

The same principle of highlighting and shading that was used to plan the application of eye shadow will be used here. To refresh your memory, refer to pages 58 and 61. The basic rule is: *light colours bring forward and make areas appear larger or more prominent; dark colours make areas recede and look smaller or less prominent.* As you were able to create illusions using light and dark shades on your eyelids and surrounding the eyes, you will here learn how to create illusions on your cheeks.

White, cream or very light colours are called highlighters. All the other colours arranged below the highlighters in the colour charts on the previous page are called shading colours. Different effects can be achieved, depending on which part of the cheek is shaded. Look at the examples on the right.

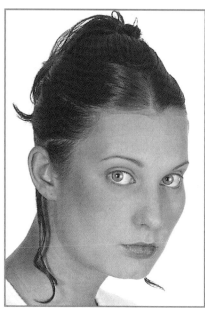

To soften a cheekbone that may already be quite prominent, the shading colour is applied along the bone itself.

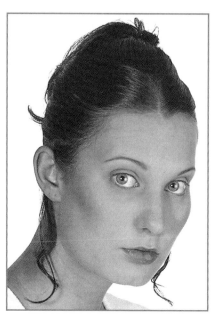

To add definition to the cheekbone or to slim the face, the shading colour is applied in a curved shape below the cheekbone.

softening a prominent cheekbone

If you feel that your cheekbones are too 'sharp' and prominent, you can 'soften' them by referring to the illustration below, and by following the steps outlined.

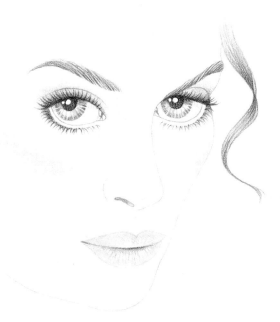

1 Simply apply a suitable shading colour (cool or warm neutral) along the cheekbone itself, as shown in the illustration on the left. This will darken the bone area, and create the illusion of it being less prominent.

2 Using a slightly larger brush, blend the colour well so that there is no hard, definite 'stripe' of colour along the cheekbone. Blending is essential to achieving a professional-looking finish.

defining a cheekbone or slimming a face

To give more definition to the cheekbone, or to slim the face, refer to the illustration below, and follow the steps outlined. The photographs refer to step 1 and step 2 only.

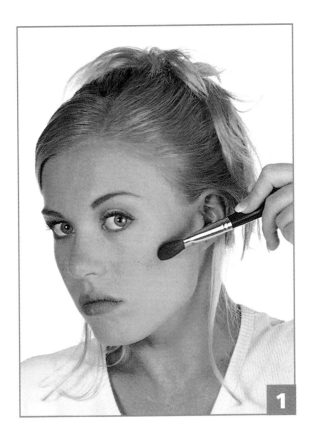

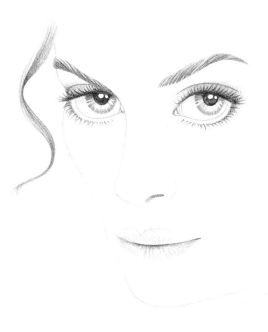

Shading is applied in a curved shape below the bone.

1 Apply a shading colour below the cheekbone, using a small, dome-shaped blusher brush.

2 Apply highlighter along the bone itself, using a slightly larger brush.

3 Now blend the 'edges' of the colours well using a clean brush. There should be no distinguishable 'bands' of colour and the presence of blusher should not be obvious in any way.

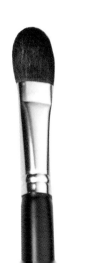

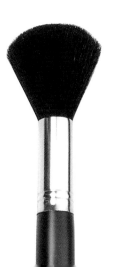

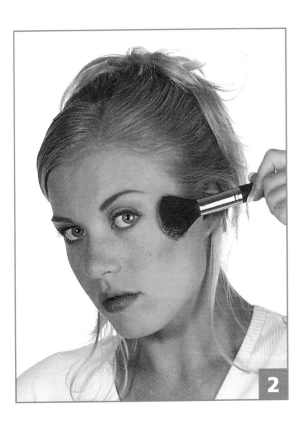

adding colour

'Colour' can be added to the face after contouring (highlighting and shading) has taken place. The best colour to choose is a very natural soft pink (marked with a ❱ in the colour chart on page 73). The pink colour should not stand out as an 'added' colour, but should look like a natural glow – as if you had just pinched your cheeks.

The colour on the immediate right is a natural pink blush, whereas the colour further to the right is too bright a pink to look natural.

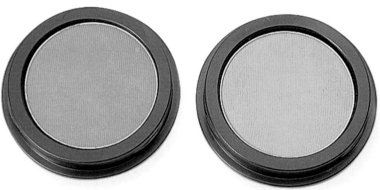

Even if you have a warm skin undertone, use a natural pink colour, as everyone goes a little pink when warm or excited. Do not think that you have to add bright orange to your cheeks to brighten your face if you have a warm skin undertone. You will, however, still be using a colour with a warm tone to it to contour your face.

If you want to add healthy-looking colour to your face – in addition to contouring – refer to the illustration and the photograph below.

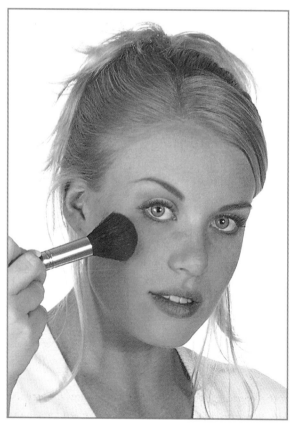

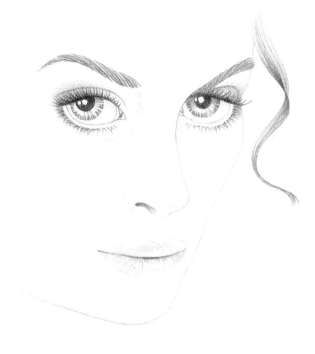

A very natural pink colour should be lightly dusted onto the cheek in the position indicated on the illustration.

the importance of positioning blusher correctly

Although the cheekbone does not slant downwards across the face in a straight line, many women apply their blusher in a straight line or 'band'. If you apply light pressure, and feel along your cheekbone, you will realize that it curves up slightly towards the front of the face. If you are applying shading colour to enhance the bone, the colour should therefore also be applied in a slight curve along the lower side of the bone, and below it.

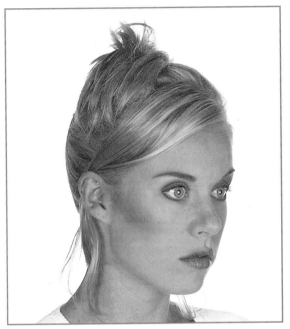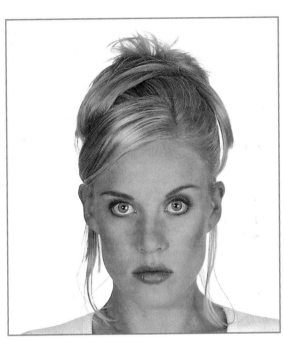

This side and front view of the same application illustrates how the contouring blusher shade correctly enhances the shape of the bone by following its natural curved shape.

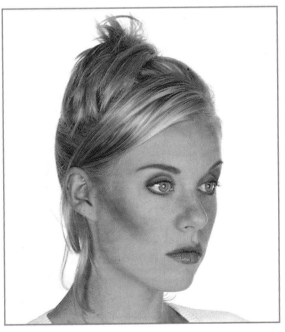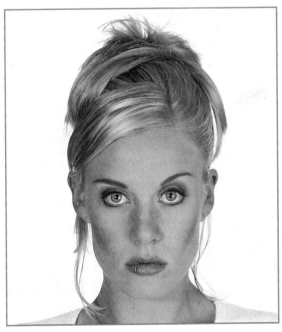

This side and front view of the same application shows how the contouring blusher shade has been incorrectly applied in a straight line. Note how the colour finishes too low towards the front of the face. It drags the shape of the face downwards and creates a 'hard' look.

lips
get the colour

Lipstick adds the finishing touch to a look by defining the mouth and adding colour to the face. It is also the step during which you can have the most fun, as there are fewer make-up 'rules' and restrictions here than anywhere else. You can transform your look in any way you like, simply by changing your lipstick colour. In a matter of seconds you can go from next-to-natural, to casual, elegant, dramatic or fun and funky. And by mixing lipsticks on the lips you can create your own unique colours.

Remember, however, that lipstick applied by itself to a face otherwise bare of make-up, will usually draw attention to any blemishes, redness or unevenness in skin tone. Examples of this effect can clearly be seen in the photographs used on pages 50 and 51. If you are applying lipstick, therefore, or changing the natural colour of your lips in any way, always ensure that your overall look is balanced. Apply foundation to even out your skin tone, and add other make-up products as well to complete your look.

decisions, decisions

Most women have the luxury of owning a variety of lipstick colours, and of being able to select a particular colour to suit a particular occasion. Your choice of colour usually depends on several factors. Firstly, you will have to determine whether you have a cool or warm skin tone, and select all your lipstick colours from either the cool or the warm palette. This is discussed in detail on pages 49–55.

Secondly, your choice of lipstick colour will be determined to some extent by the colours of the clothing you are wearing. Your lipstick colour should not clash with your outfit, for example, but complement it. If you are wearing a smart red blazer for a business meeting, for instance, an application of an equally strong red lipstick can be highly effective and communicate your confidence.

The last factor to consider is the style of dress, in terms of casual daily wear or smart evening attire. If you are wearing casual jeans and a T-shirt, I would recommend a natural lip colour rather than a deep burgundy, for instance. On the other hand, if you are wearing an evening gown, strong, dark lip colours may be preferable to pale peach or pearly pink. Refer to the photographs of the glamorous evening look created on page 67, for example, or to the section on fun and funky looks for the young on pages 86–87.

lipstick colours

Many make-up houses do not separate their cool and warm colours for display purposes, so you will have to use your own judgement to categorize a lipstick as either cool or warm. (Cool and warm colours are discussed in detail on pages 48–57.)

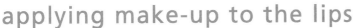

Before purchasing lipstick, test the colour on the back of your hand. Ask yourself whether you can see more pink or mauve tones in the colour, or whether you can see more orange and yellow tones. If you see more pink or mauve tones, the colour is cool; if you can see more orange or yellow tones, it is a warm colour.

The lipstick colour chart reproduced on page 80 illustrates just some of the many colours I would recommend, both from the cool and the warm palette.

applying make-up to the lips

There are several products and several techniques involved in applying make-up to the lips in a professional way. It is important to know why and how each product is used, and why, when and how certain techniques are applied. Treat your lips well, as chapped, dry or flaky lips can be a nightmare to work with.

moisturizing dry lips

If your lips are dry, first soften them by applying a lip balm and allowing it a few minutes to soak into the skin. Then blot the lips on a tissue to remove excess oiliness.

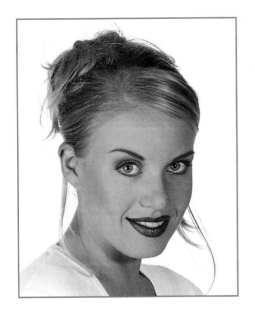

If you have been brave enough to buy a very different colour to what you are used to wearing, experiment over weekends. Apply the lip colour while you are at home, and look at yourself in the mirror every now and again. By doing this, you will gradually 'train' your eye to like it.

Your lipstick application technique can 'make or break' your look. Whether you opt for a natural or dark lipstick colour, aim to achieve a balanced overall effect.

lipstick colours

cool

warm

choosing lipstick colours

Once you have narrowed down your selection of colours, *try them on your lips* to test the colour properly. The same lipstick used by a friend may well produce a different colour on your own lips. You may need to go out of the store to check the colour in natural light, as fluorescent light can distort your perception of the true colour.

The colours reproduced on this page are only a small selection of the endless variety available. They are intended merely as a guide to either the cool or the warm shades that may suit you. If you struggle to choose colours when faced with the array at the cosmetics counter, you may want to take this book along to guide you.

key

+ not recommended for small lips

If your lip pencil is not exactly the same colour as your lipstick, use a lipstick brush or cotton bud to smudge the pencilled line inwards towards the centre of the mouth so that the two colours blend effectively.

lining the lips

Use a lip pencil in the same colour as the lipstick or in a slightly darker colour. The qualities of a good lip pencil are discussed on page 24. The pencil should be sharpened and any scratchy edges can then be softened slightly on a tissue.

When lining your lips, do not simply start along the upper lip and work you way round the mouth, following the natural lip edge. If you want to correct any 'faults' in terms of lip shape – and very few people have perfectly symmetrical mouths – it will be easier to do on a mouth bare of colour. The easiest way to balance the appearance of your lips whilst lining, is to divide the mouth into sections, and work on each part in turn until the lines are connected.

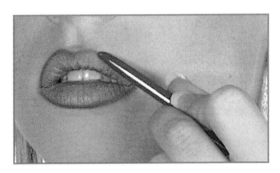

Follow the numbering in the illustration below – and the corresponding text – to learn the correct sequence when pencilling.

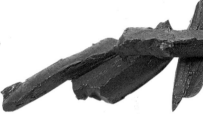

1 Start in the middle of the upper lip, and line the Cupid's bow as shown. You will immediately be able to see where other sections of your lips may be uneven.

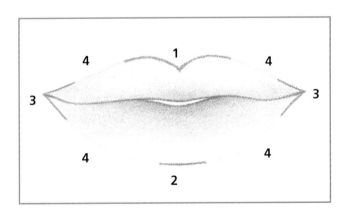

2 Now move to the centre of your bottom lip, and draw a short, horizontal line.

3 The next step is to line the corners of your mouth. If your lips are asymmetric, refer to the illustration at the bottom of this page. If your lips are close to symmetrical, carefully draw in two neat corners.

4 Finally, connect the lines drawn in the centre (top and bottom) to the corners.

correcting the lip shape

If your lips are irregular or asymmetric in shape, as illustrated below, it is possible to create the illusion of almost perfectly balanced lips when lining your lips with pencil.

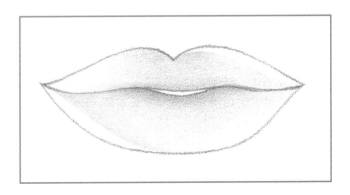

1 Follow the same sequence set out above for lining uneven lips. Line the centres of your lips first, before moving to the corners.

2 Create the illusion of balance between your top and bottom lips by 'correcting' your lip shape subtly, ensuring that your pencilled lines meet precisely at the corners. In this example, both the upper and lower lips have been 'corrected' in terms of shape.

applying lipstick

1 Use a small, firm lipstick brush of sable hair (see page 13) to apply lipstick. Work carefully, creating a smooth, clean edge. If you apply lipstick straight from the tube, you will never achieve a perfect edge, and you will need to re-apply lipstick more frequently.

2 Blot your lips on a tissue and apply a second coat.

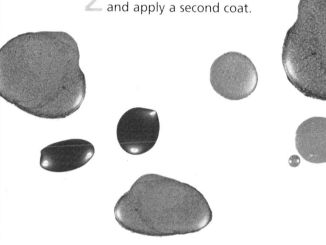

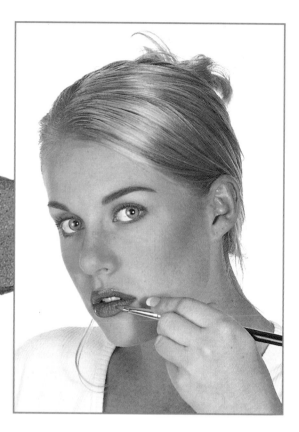

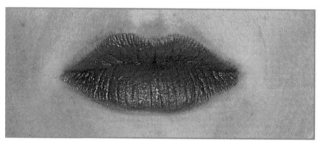

Take great care when applying lipstick in dark colours, as any of the following common mistakes will be more obvious.

Left: *Avoid irregular lip edges like these, which look really messy.*

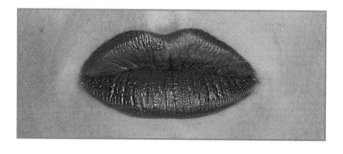

Left: *Take care not to work too far out beyond the natural edge. This will only make it obvious that you would prefer having fuller lips. Also refer to page 81, in terms of 'correcting' the lip shape.*

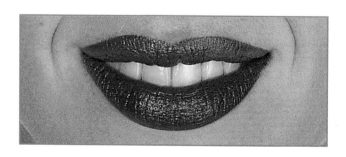

Left: *Edges should be clean and neat, following the natural lip line as closely as possible.*

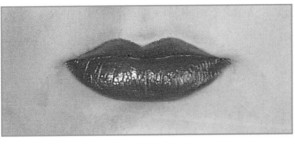

Here a smaller top lip has been filled in incorrectly, and the corners do not look balanced (refer to the discussion of asymmetric lips on page 81).

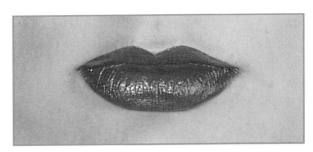

The corners of the top lip have now been correctly filled out to meet those of the bottom lip, creating an illusion of balance. The look is still perfectly natural.

applying lip gloss

Lips high on gloss tend to come and go as a make-up trend, so keep an eye on the fashions of the time. Lip gloss is applied after lipstick, and then only to the centre of lips. Applied close to the edge of your lips, lip gloss tends to 'bleed' beyond the lip edges. If your lipstick tends to bleed in any case, avoid adding lip gloss. Mature skins, especially, should avoid using lip gloss.

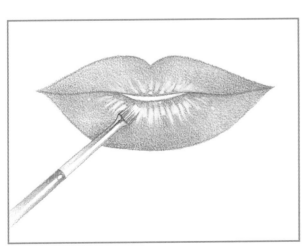

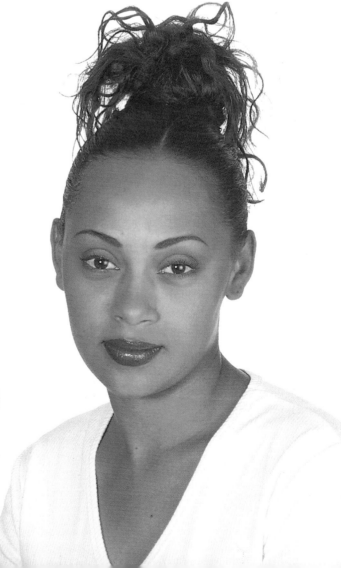

Above and right: Apply lip gloss to the centre of the lips only, to avoid lipstick bleeding beyond the edges of the lip line. Here lip gloss is also used to enhance attractive, full lips.

colour that lasts

If you want your lipstick application to last as long as possible without re-application being necessary, I recommend using matte lipstick. Several layers of lipstick can be applied, and lips should be blotted on a tissue before each new layer is applied.

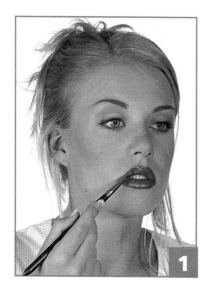

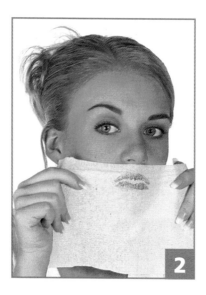

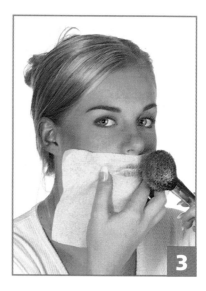

1 Apply matte lipstick, which usually lasts longer than any other kind.

2 After applying one layer of lipstick, gently blot the lips on a tissue.

3 Then apply a light dusting of loose powder through the tissue.

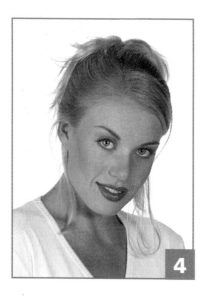

4 Apply a final layer of lipstick, but do not apply powder over it.

Unfortunately, the longer you want your lipstick to last, the dryer the lipstick has to be, and this can begin to feel uncomfortable. A creamier lipstick will keep your lips softer, but, owing to the added moisture in the lipstick, it will not last as long. There is no happy medium here. If you want lip colour that lasts, you have to sacrifice the comfort of soft lips. If you want soft, comfortable lips, you will have to sacrifice staying power.

mature skin

As one ages, your colouring in terms of skin, lips, eyes and hair changes subtly. This means that colours that may have looked great on your face at twenty, may no longer be flattering at thirty or forty. The colours may be too strong for your skin tone or too pale to add colour to a face that needs more brightening than it used to.

When it comes to choosing lipstick colours, pale, frosted or pearly shades should be avoided completely. These are the least flattering on mature skin. Also avoid lip gloss.

The most common problem in the case of mature skin, is that of lipstick 'bleeding' or spreading outwards from the lips into the fine lines around the mouth. To help prevent this, follow the steps outlined below, and study the photographs.

1 Use a high-quality lip pencil – not soft and smudgy – to neatly define the outline of your lips. In addition to lining the lips, also use the pencil to shade the lips lightly.

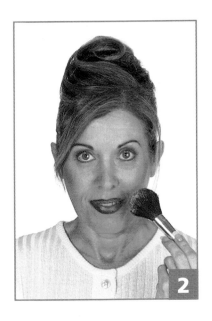

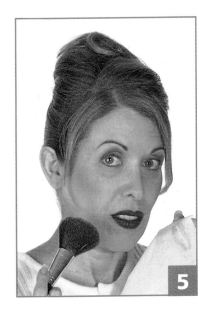

2 Apply loose powder to the entire shaded area, and then apply a *matte* lipstick. (These lipsticks are drier and less creamy and will therefore not bleed as easily).

3 Gently press the lips onto a tissue to blot.

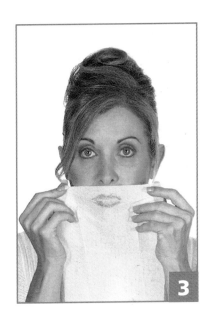

4 Lightly dust loose powder onto the lips through the tissue, using a powder brush.

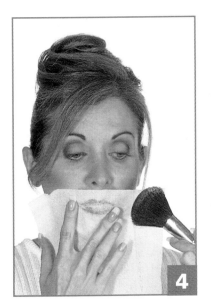

5 Repeat the process set out here two to three times, finishing with an application of loose powder.

over the top

There is always a time and a place just for having fun – and where almost no make-up 'rules' apply. An adventurous night on the town provides a perfect opportunity to delight your fancy in the latest fashion fads. Add sparkle and colour – the more the better. Shine and shimmer to your heart's content. Wow the crowds who go clubbing and outshine the dance floor's lights!

breaking all the rules

As many regular clubbers will agree, half the fun of the party lies in planning and preparing your look. The other half is enjoying showing off what you have accomplished. Now is the time to break all the rules, and make use of the enormous variety of fun products. And make-up application is certainly not limited to the face alone – use it on shoulders, collarbones, and even on your hair. Body paint is fun and funky, and you can keep everyone guessing by applying a little temporary 'tattoo' in the form of a cheeky transfer or stencilled shape.

shimmer dust or glitter dust is a loose, fine eye-shadow powder with a high shimmer or sparkle content that 'lights up' as light strikes it. The powder colour will determine its positioning. Gold and pearl can be dusted virtually anywhere; pinks and mauves are great for cheeks or eyes, but green and blue are best kept for the eyes. Use a brush, tapping off excess powder onto a tissue, and lightly dust only a small amount of powder on at a time.

a pearlized finish can be achieved by using a pearlized foundation or cream in stick form. This can be applied lightly over the entire face – and body – using a latex sponge. It is very effective to highlight specific areas like cheekbones and browbones.

glitter gel is one of the easiest and quickest ways of transforming any look to suit the club. It can be used anywhere on the face or body, over or without other make-up products, and it is available in a variety of colours. Usually one finds a clear gel base, carrying coloured glitter. Coloured glitter gel consists of a *coloured* gel base carrying glitter. This provides instant colour as well as glitter – a wonderful substitute for eye shadow.

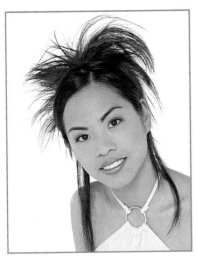

Here dark green shadow creates evening eyes. Lips are kept quite natural, only given a pearly finish.

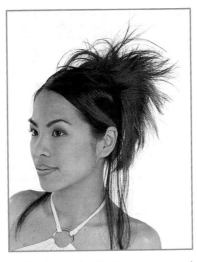

Gold dust highlights brows and cheekbones. Blue and green face paint make for 'mermaid' lips.

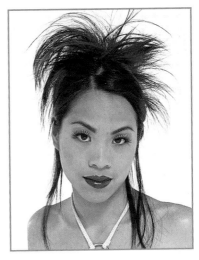

Go over the top with false lashes in metallic green. Strengthen the mouth with plummy lip gloss.

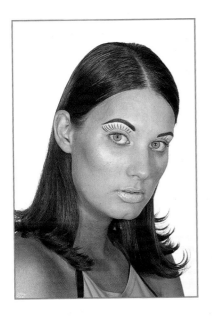

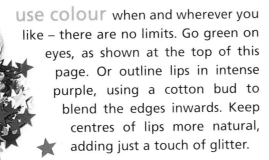

face paint or eye paint can be used to add bold, fun colours and dramatic painted shapes. Seen under flashing lights, the effect is striking. Icy pastel shades combine well with strong colours.

brightly coloured hair can easily be achieved using coloured hair mascara or spray. Use fluorescent colours on very dark hair, and almost anything but gold on blonde hair – then simply wash the colour out.

stick-on shapes can be applied by just using a little petroleum jelly as an adhesive. Add a few stars to a cheek or temple, or develop your own design.

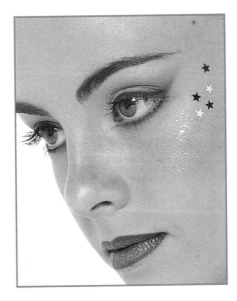

use colour when and wherever you like – there are no limits. Go green on eyes, as shown at the top of this page. Or outline lips in intense purple, using a cotton bud to blend the edges inwards. Keep centres of lips more natural, adding just a touch of glitter.

literally, almost anything goes . . .

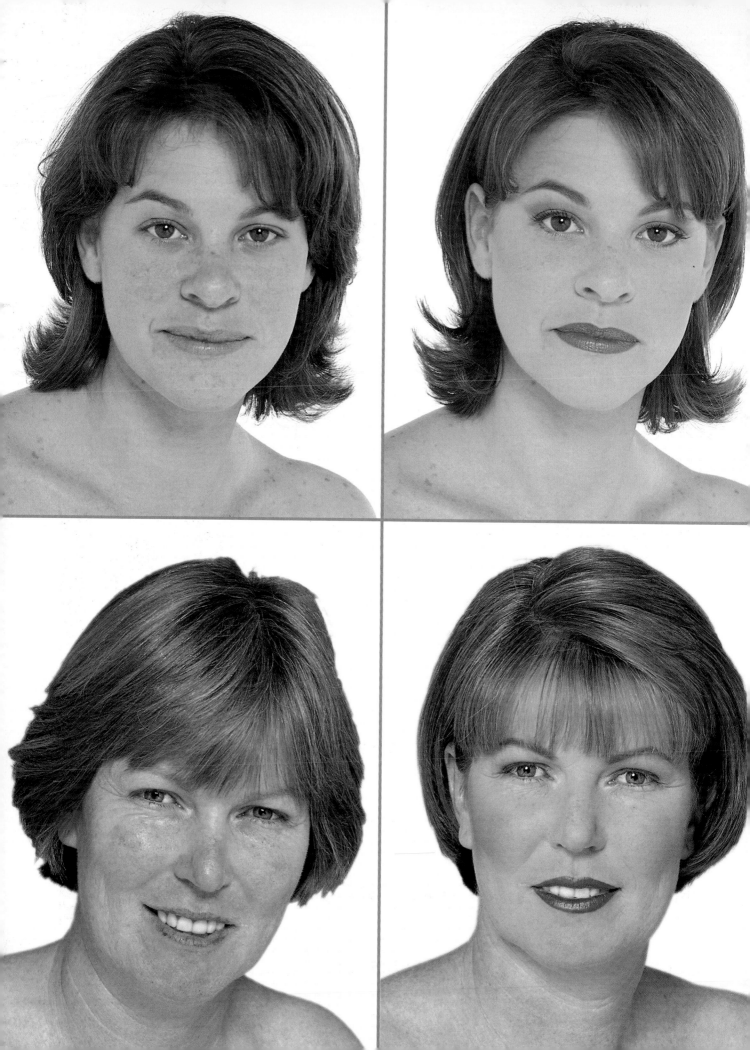

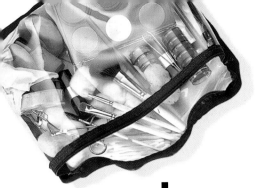

make-overs

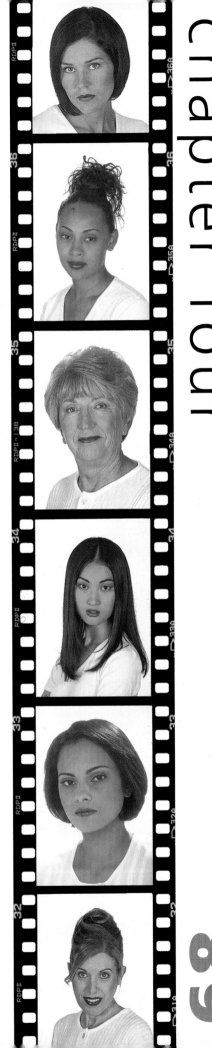

Whether your goal is simply to update your look a little, or to create an entirely new image, this chapter is offered as a source of inspiration. Though some of these transformations may seem like magic, there are no hidden tricks. If you allow yourself to be guided by what you see in this book, there is no reason why you cannot create looks like these yourself.

make-overs
make magic

During my career as a professional make-up artist and teacher, scores of women have consulted me about changing and enhancing their looks. All too often, though, before I have had a chance to say anything, they have also already told me what kind of look they *do not* want.

It is a fact that we all grow used to and comfortable with seeing ourselves looking a particular way. We react with shock when we suddenly see our comfortable image having been altered by a hairstylist, for instance. Or we balk at the mere suggestion of trying something altogether different. We feel that we know ourselves better than anyone else, and are therefore able to judge better than anyone else what suits us and what does not.

The truth is that we are very rarely able to look at ourselves objectively. It is important, therefore, when considering a change, not to defend against suggestions immediately. If you are consulting a professionally trained make-up artist or hairstylist, listen carefully to their ideas. Their advice will be based on their professional opinion – informed by their training, expertise and experience.

Practise using your judgement by studying the two photographs on this page, and deciding which make-up application enhances the face most, creating a younger, fresher appearance.

which is better?

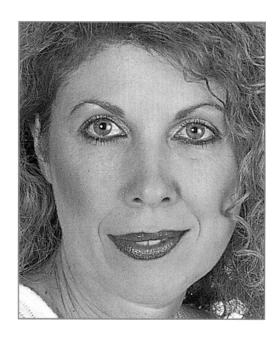 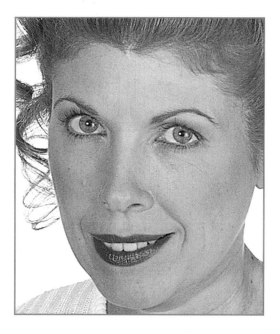

shimmer eye shadow?
coloured products, like eye shadow?
dark, pencilled eyeliner?
hard, strong blusher?
glossy lipstick?

or

subtle, matte eye shadow?
neutral eye shadow and other products?
smoky, blended shadow as eyeliner?
soft, natural blusher?
matte lipstick?

making the change & sticking with it

Even if you feel uncomfortable with a new look at first and immediately want to revert to what you are used to, decide to give your new image a chance. Do not restyle your hair or wash off all your make-up the minute you reach home. Ask yourself whether you really know what suits you best, or whether you just know what you have become used to. After a few weeks of 'bearing with' your new style of make-up or haircut, you may find yourself wondering why you did not change before.

The information provided in this book gives you the key to looking great – anywhere, and anytime. No matter what your colouring, your age or your lifestyle – you will always look your best in 'nearly natural', neutral, matte make-up. Look at the variety of women included in this chapter.

I sincerely hope that this series of make-overs inspires you to use the art of make-up to make the most of yourself – always.

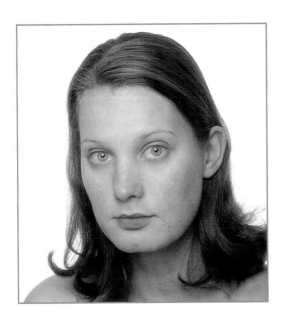

before   after

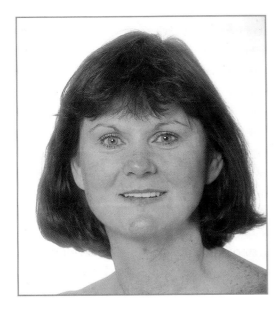

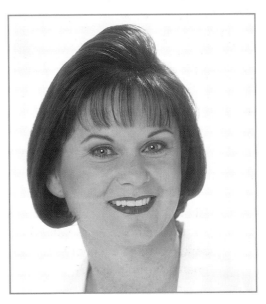

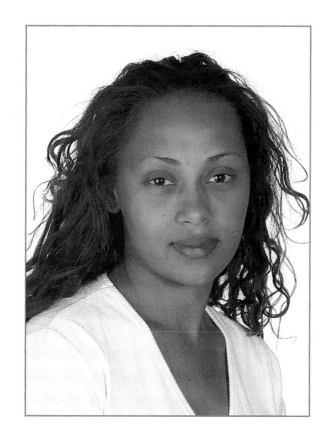

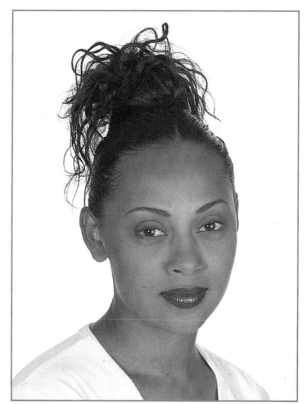

before

after

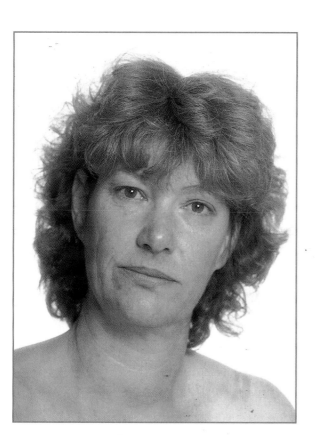

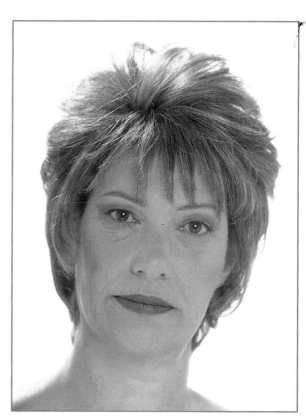

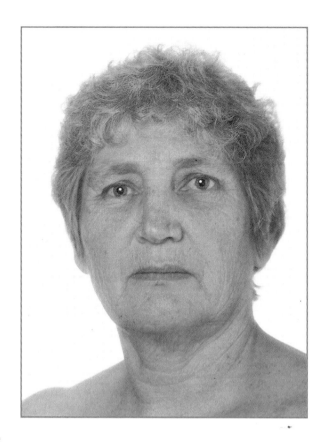

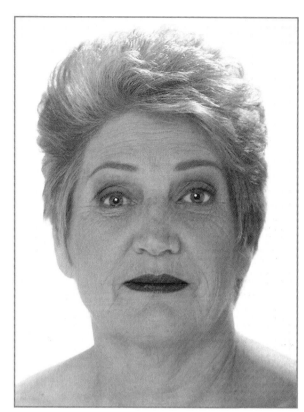

before   after

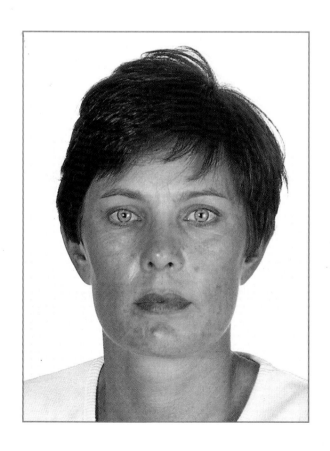

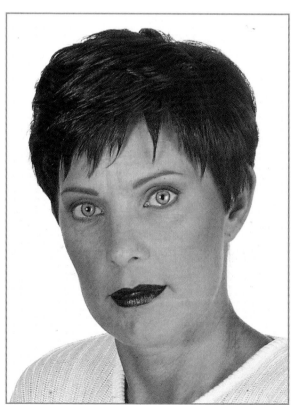

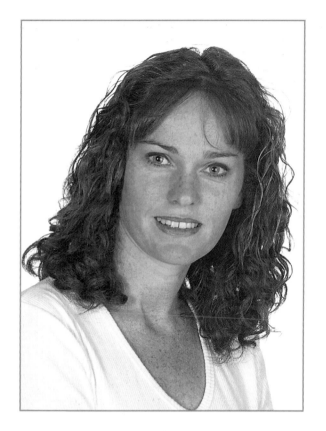

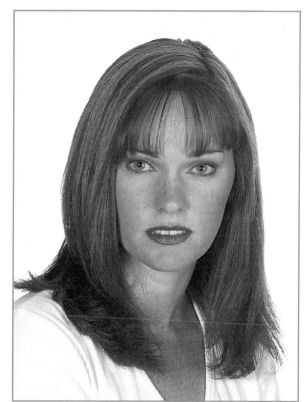

before   after

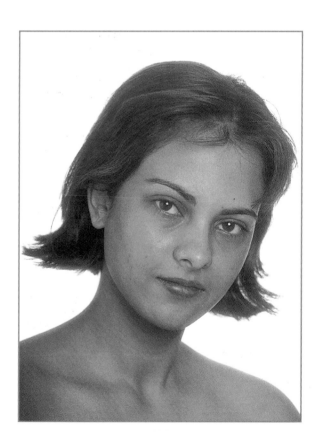

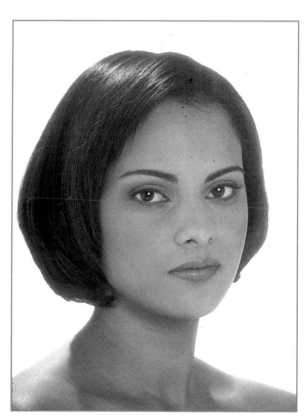

Most of the products and equipment discussed in this book are available from large pharmacies and department stores with good cosmetics counters. Some readers who may not live near a major centre, however, may experience difficulty in obtaining certain items. These readers are encouraged to contact a professional supplier closest to their area, selected from the list provided below. These suppliers do not deal only with professional make-up artist but can be very helpful to anyone seriously interested in the art of make-up, or in obtaining a particular product or accessory.

Alcone Co
549 49th Avenue
Long Island City
NY 11101-5610, USA
Tel: (718) 361 8373
Mail-order suppliers for make-up of all brands.

California Theatrical Supply
132 9th Street
San Francisco
CA 94103-2603, USA
Tel: (415) 863 923
Distributors of Kryolan make-up to the West Coast of the USA.

Charles H Fox Ltd
22 Tavistock Street, Covent Garden
London WC2E 7PY
England
Tel: (020) 7240 3111

Cinema Secrets
4400 West Riverside Drive
Burbank
CA 91505-4097, USA
Tel: (818) 563 9213
Suppliers of a full line of professional make-up products.

Cosmetics a la Carte Ltd
Unit 102, Avro House
Havelock Terrace
London SW8 4AS
England
Tel/Fax: (020) 7622 2318
Website: www.a-la-carte.co.uk
Suppliers of a full line of professional make-up, specializing in hard-to-find colours. Free brochure and full mail-order service of products and equipment, as well as a studio to visit for individual lessons or practical advice.

Frends Beauty Supply Co
5270 Laurel Canyon Boulevard
North Hollywood
CA 91607-2792, USA
Tel: (818) 769 3834

Joe Blasco Cosmetics
1670 Hillhurst Ave # 202-3
Los Angeles
CA 90027-5580, USA
Suppliers of the full Joe Blasco Cosmetic line.

Kryolan Corp
132 9th Street
San Francisco
CA 94103-2603
USA
Tel: (415) 863 9236
Suppliers of a full line of theatrical make-up.

Make-up Center Ltd
150 West 55th Street
New York City
NY 10019-5305
USA
Tel: (212) 997 9494

Make Up For Ever
Hyde Park Corner
Jan Smuts Avenue
Johannesburg
South Africa
Tel: (011) 325 5035

Josie Knowland
Film Make Up Technology
5 The Crescent
Annandale
NSW 2038
Australia
Tel: (02) 9518 9000

Make Up For Ever
Sandton City Shopping Centre
Sandton
Johannesburg
South Africa
Tel: (011) 883 7091

The Make-up School (Cape Town)
P.O. Box 6672
Welgemoed
7538
South Africa
Tel: (021) 910 4150

The Make-up School (Johannesburg)
P.O. Box 1877
Rivonia
2128
South Africa
Tel: (011) 807 2844
Full nationwide mail-order service for products and equipment, as well as professional training and individual make-up classes.

Naimie's Beauty Center
12640 Riverside Drive
North Hollywood
CA 91607-3411, USA
Tel: (818) 655 9933
Fax: (818) 655 9999
Website: www.naimies.com
Professional suppliers of over 50 different brands of make-up and accessories.

Professional Make-up
Cavendish Square
Cavendish Street
Claremont
South Africa
Tel: (021) 671 3344

Professional Make-up
Tyger Valley Centre
Willie van Schoor Avenue
Bellville, South Africa
Tel: (021) 914 3410

Screenface
24 Powis Terrace, London
W11 1JH, England
Tel: (020) 7221 8289
and
48 Monmouth Street, London
WC2H 9EP, England
Tel: (020) 7836 3955
Suppliers of a full line of all professional make-up products and accessories.

There are now various salons throughout South Africa that stock Professional Make-up products. As these details constantly change (salons move or new salons arise), we have introduced an information line whereby readers from all over the country can call to enquire about a stockist in their area. For more information, please call (0860) 10 21 25.

To obtain further information on the availability of quality make-up tools or products, write to the author:

Joy Terri
P.O. Box 6672
Welgemoed
7538
South Africa

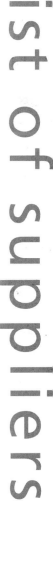

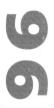

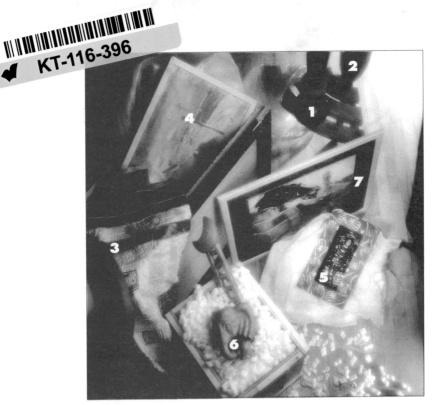

Cover photograph

The work illustrated on the cover was kindly lent by the artists below. Many thanks to Denise Henderson, Terry McCartney and Martin Senior from the Northern Centre for Contemporary Art, Sunderland, for their assistance with the cover. Cover photograph by Colin Cuthbert.
See photo for numerical key to artists' work.

1   Glass vase by **Stuart Akroyd**, Frederick Street Studios, 52 Back Frederick Street, Sunderland SR1 1NA tel 091 510 1377

2   *The Fish Chair,* by **Keith Ashford**, 18 Derwentdale Gardens, High Heaton, Newcastle tel 091 281 2769

3   Embroidered tapestry by **Julie Heppell**, 22 Mandarin Lodge, Felling, Gateshead tel 091 469 8015

4   Landscape, oil on canvas, by **Alan McGinn**, 53 Front Street, East Boldon, Tyne & Wear NE38 0SH tel 091 519 2275 (collection David Butler)

5   *Come on in out of the dark*, papier maché relief wooden box by **Cath Rive**, 3 Thornhill Gardens, Sunderland SR2 7LD tel 091 510 1820

6   *It's OK to make mistakes,* polychrome wood, by **Chris Sell**, 1 St Bedes Terrace, Sunderland SR2 8HS tel 091 565 3402 (collection Susan Jones and Richard Padwick)

7   *The end of the road,* photomontage by **Nicky Taylor**, Burn Cottage, 1 Noble Terrace, Sunderland SR2 8LX (collection Helen Smith)

Acknowledgements

I would like to thank all the artists and organisations who so willingly contributed information and shared their experiences of selling and exhibiting abroad. Particular thanks are due to Jenny Beavan, Jane Adam, Trisha Clarke, Ken Devine, Les Buckingham of Aspex Gallery, Mark Goldsworthy, Annie Doherty, Juliette Goddard, Emma Sewell, Clare Henshaw, Roshini Kempadoo, Rhonda Wilson, Carole Waller, Jonathan Andersson, Neil Bottle, Nick Allen, Rob Turner and others whose work is illustrated in the book. Thanks also to Hilary Strong of Natural Theatre for information on carnets, Louise Scott of IETM for inspiration on networking and Sue Webber of Bristol Chamber of Commerce for exporting advice. The quote from Alasdair MacDonell in Chapter 1 is from *Ceramic Review*.

Writer

Judith Staines is the author of *Making Connections: a craftsperson's guide to Europe* (South West Arts) and *Selling* (AN Publications). As a freelance arts consultant she undertakes research and cultural project management for arts boards and other bodies.

Note

All prices quoted and services mentioned in this book are believed to be accurate at the time of going to press (April 94). But any readers exhibiting and selling abroad should always check specific information at the time they need it. Customs regulations, in particular, can change without warning.

Contents

Contents

Artists Handbooks
Exhibiting & Selling Abroad

by
Judith Staines

AN Publications

By giving access to information, advice and debate, AN Publications aims to:

- empower artists individually and collectively to strengthen their professional position
- raise awareness of the diversity of visual arts practice and encourage an equality of opportunity
- stimulate good working practices throughout the visual arts.

Series Editor	David Butler
Readers	Jane Adam, Richard Murphy and Caroline Douglas
Proof reader	Heather Cawte Winskill (100 Proof)
Index	Susanne Atkin
Cover photograph	Colin Cuthbert
Design & layout	Neil Southern
Grant aid	Arts Council of England and Crafts Council
Printer	Mayfair Printers, Commercial Road, Hendon, Sunderland SR2 8NP
Copyright	The writers, photographers and Artic Producers Publishing Co Ltd © 1994

ISBN 0 907730 21 3

**AN Publications is an imprint of
Artic Producers Publishing Co Ltd
PO Box 23, Sunderland SR4 6DG tel 091 567 3589**

1 • Boats & bees

Before the fall of the Berlin Wall artist Mark Thompson created an installation which made a powerful statement about the nature of political frontiers and the ability of art to cross them. Built at the Kunstlerhaus Bethanien, the work included a swarm of West German bees which flew freely around East and West Berlin, returning to the gallery with pollen collected from both sides.

Since then, the Wall has come down, new borders have been drawn and there is free movement of goods within the European Union. But even now, most artworks don't cross borders under their own steam.

This is a book for all artists and makers who want to promote themselves and their work overseas. It takes a broad interpretation of 'exporting' to include exhibiting and residencies abroad, as well as selling in a range of situations. Exporting here means any activity that involves artworks or artists crossing borders.

International mobility is the key to success and satisfaction for many artists and makers. What motivates them? It may be commercial success or the knowledge that international networking is essential to their artistic creation.

All artists and makers who are now experienced exporters describe the steep learning curve they had to tackle when they first started exporting. Information and advice specific to their needs was hard to find. So this book sets out to bridge that gap with practical information, reassurance and plenty of examples of artists and makers who have done it. It describes the whole range of exporting experience, from the simplest ways of getting work from A to B to very much more complex shipping methods and payment arrangements.

British artists can suffer from a degree of insularity. With a land border with only one other country, the UK does still embody a spirit of isolation which is apparent in its relations with mainland Europe and other parts of the world.

Historically the UK developed its strongest trading relationships with far-flung colonies. In the 1990s, government approaches to exporting, which speak of 'conquering overseas markets', still seem tainted by a desire for colonisation.

Are the government agencies which promote overseas trade equipped to respond to the needs of artists and makers? One Customs officer, when asked for the export documentation required for a small craft business, replied: "What size boat are you talking about?"

It's also likely that business agencies may not understand the scale you are working on. When economic assistance for 'small and medium sized enterprises' is targeted at businesses employing up to 250 people, self-employed artists and makers (who are mainly one-person businesses) find they come pretty low down on the priority list. A government export credit guarantee scheme, which offers insurance against overseas buyers who don't pay their bills, is designed for businesses with an export turnover of at least £50,000.

So there is a lack of encouragement and support which is confirmed by the comparatively low level of participation by UK artists and makers in international competitions.

And yet the quality of work made by artists in the UK is exceptionally high by world standards. The strength of our art and design education is widely recognised. In a recent survey, Britain was found to have far more colleges of higher education teaching craft and design courses than other European countries.

The benefits of working and thinking internationally are apparent in the confidence and openness of artists who successfully promote themselves overseas. It gives them a breadth of vision and a stronger base for earning their living as an artist.

One of the ways of achieving this is through international networking among artists. Describing the isolation of Swiss artists, Anne Biéler, President of Informal European Theatre Meeting, perhaps the most effective European network of cultural organisations, stressed that "mobility is a state of mind". However isolated you are geographically, culturally or politically, if you think internationally, you can experience the freedom to move across borders. International networking can help you understand the different contexts in which artists work.

Experience of exporting

"I find that once you are across the Channel, there aren't any barriers." **Trisha Clarke, painter**

"Exporting is brilliant. The orders are larger than for the UK and I don't get asked to do sale or return." **Sally Penn Smith, glass designer**

"Exporting is totally daunting at first but you soon get used to it. The UK is a very limited market so you've got to look elsewhere." **Neil Bottle, textile designer**

"People really love art in Switzerland and there's a tradition of building up a relationship between the artist and buyer. It's a very forward-looking society." **Juliette Goddard, painter**

"Leaving America ... confident that there is a huge market there and a receptivity to ideas that fall outside the conventions that often seem to inhibit British ceramics. This journey has given me enormous insight and useful knowledge." **Alasdair MacDonell, ceramicist**

"There are some beautiful galleries in mainland Europe. The work looks good, the publicity is high quality and collectors take the work more seriously." **Clare Henshaw, glass artist**

"In my experience, 90% of things happen through artists. Almost all my overseas exhibitions have come about through networking, exchanging information and recommendations. The way you start to make contact with artists in other countries is through common issues in the work." **Susan Derges, photographer**

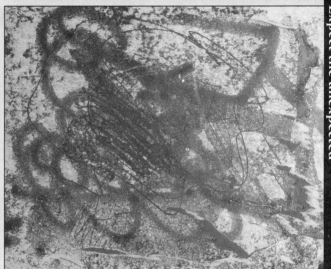

Trisha Clarke,
First tear, **36" x
24", etching.
Photo:** the artist

Trisha Clarke is a London-based artist. In 1989 she and a partner formed an art consultancy called EuroArt to promote artists and their work in Europe.

In 1991 Trisha decided to organise a show in Paris. The first step was to identify the right gallery and establish a partnership. They visited Paris and viewed a number of galleries. Finding the right place involved presenting the proposal to the gallery owner, negotiating a budget and securing an agreement. The result was a contract with Galerie Oz to co-curate an exhibition called 'London Look' in 1992 featuring Trisha's paintings and sculpture by Anthony-Noel Kelly.

They transported work to Paris themselves in a borrowed van. The show was on for a month, received favourable reviews and a good percentage of work sold. There were unexpected successes too. During the private view a passer-by who stopped for a look turned out to be the Art Director of a major music publishing group. He negotiated a copyright licence on two works by Trisha for use as CD covers. The contract detailed different geographical markets, the scale of charges for a limited number of reproductions with royalty fees beyond this edition. The original paintings sold during the exhibition as well. However, the return in copyright licence fees and royalties has now exceeded the selling price of the paintings.

In November 1992 EuroArt mounted another exhibition, this time in Cadiz in Southern Spain. The gallery,

Arte Elemental, was recommended by an artist and contact with the gallery owner secured an exhibition agreement. Here there was a more straightforward commercial arrangement. The gallery paid for publicity, invitations, private view and took a commission of 35% on works sold. As organisers EuroArt agreed a commission on works sold with selected artists who were individually responsible for arranging insurance of their works.

Work was transported to Cadiz as a part-load by Prima European, a general removals firm who packed and crated work under the supervision of EuroArt. Trisha found them through the *Costa Blanca News* (an English language newspaper for expatriates living in Spain) and said the service was excellent, costing just £150 per artist.

Trisha attended the private view, a lively 8 hour event complete with Spanish dancers. The selection of very colourful work was, she felt, essential for the strong Southern light and local visual taste. Again the unexpected happened. November, which they were warned would be a quiet time for visitors and sales, turned out to be ideal for local people who avoid galleries during the busy tourist season. It's also a time for refitting businesses and seven pieces sold to two restaurants being redesigned.

A surprise visitor to the exhibition was a German gallery owner who offered to show Trisha's unsold work at his gallery in the Kreishaus district of Cologne where there are several good art galleries. The show would coincide with the Kölner Kunsttage (the Cologne Art Day), an annual event jointly promoted by the city's galleries. He organised and paid for transport and sold work on a 50% commission basis. After exhibiting the paintings for six weeks, the gallery kept the paintings for a further three months before the remaining unsold work was returned to London in a British theatre company's van. The gallery owner knew the theatre director and made the arrangements while the company was performing in Cologne. As Trisha says, "I find that once you are across the Channel, there aren't any barriers."

EuroArt are planning a Berlin exhibition and will visit galleries there in 1994 to make contacts and identify the right place. Trisha feels it's essential to the success of any exhibiting venture to see the space for yourself. She also stresses the importance of languages and networking with other independent curators in Europe.

2 • Why export?

Any business publication will give you a number of classic reasons for exporting. Survival is usually the first, closely followed by the need to develop a range of markets (to avoid relying exclusively on one place), gaining new markets for seasonal products, and meeting competition in a global market.

The desire to work internationally, to be appreciated, exhibited, purchased and acclaimed internationally is a driving force among many artists. But when you talk to visual artists about why they want to export and promote their work internationally, a new set of reasons emerges. In fact, the starting point may simply be 'Why not?'

Certainly business concerns and the need to survive economically are likely to be a motivating factor. Makers are generally aware that they work in a competitive, commercial environment. Their approach to pricing and selling is strongly influenced by market conditions. This is frequently what drives them to look beyond the UK and develop outlets in other countries. In contrast, fine artists are initially more likely to be drawn into the business of exporting out of a desire to promote their work internationally through exhibitions. For them selling work may be a secondary and more peripheral issue.

Whatever the first reason for starting to export, and it is worth noting that most artists and makers begin by default rather than intent, there are a number of common factors which sustain the activity. It is useful to explore these.

An international community of artists

Making art can be a solitary business. Artists continue to work in isolation and are aware of being thinly dispersed in society. Even where studio groups form there is a sense of being on the edge. The opportunity to relate to artists in other countries offers a real sense of becoming part of the international community of artists.

Language is not necessarily a problem since artists share broadly similar concerns and can relate their experience directly to that of artists in other countries. There is a genuine excitement at finding like-minded people elsewhere in the world who understand what you are doing and why you persevere at it.

Lidija Kolovrat, a Croatian artist living in Lisbon, was delighted to be put in touch with a British artist who, like her, paints fabric and makes clothes which are on the borders of conceptual art and fashion. "After all," she said, "we are a very small family of artists doing this in the world. We need to find each other."

International status

The second key motivation for working internationally is the perceived value of an international reputation. Once you have had a number of exhibitions in other countries (which you can list on your CV and for which you can produce catalogues and press cuttings), galleries, potential purchasers and funding bodies in the UK are liable to show more interest in your work. Of course some international galleries are well known and an exhibition in a public museum or gallery will carry more weight than a show in a little-known commercial gallery or shop. But it must be acknowledged that few people have a detailed knowledge of the standing of galleries in a wide range of countries.

At a certain level therefore, artists can be confident that showing evidence of 'an international reputation' will stand them in good stead. However, this is not encouragement to naively pursue anything international in a tokenistic fashion. As with all investments of time and money, there has to be a real value and interest for the artist. A bad exhibiting experience is a bad experience, whether it's in London, New York or Paris, and in the long run is not likely to help your career.

Business survival international

Developing international markets is a valid and increasingly necessary means of survival for many artists. Selling work in the UK is not always easy. You may find that other countries offer more opportunities in terms of outlets, a greater inclination to purchase contemporary work

Les Bicknell, *a book of blank maps with instructions*, **1994, a book work – letterpress type folded paper**

Book artist Les Bicknell exhibited at the Frankfurt Book Fair in 1992. He shared a stand with fellow book artist Matthew Tyson who has shown there for many years. For Les it was an extremely rewarding experience: "It was wonderful! There are so few of us in this country and people don't know what a book artist is. At Frankfurt I met a whole international community of book artists – even some from the UK I didn't know – as well as collectors who understood what I did and wanted to buy the work. My wife and I went so the cost of stand, travel and accommodation was around £1,000. I went there to meet people and talk about book art – we didn't actually expect to make money but in fact we sold around £3,000 worth of work. By the end I started buying art myself and swapping work with other book artists. The follow up since then has been several private sales and I supply work to a US bookshop which sells book art."

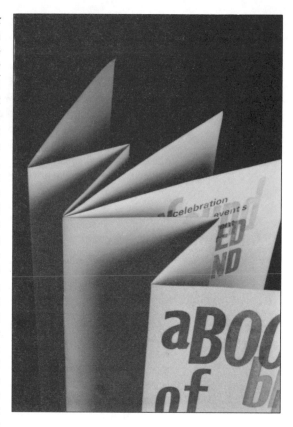

and a real understanding and appreciation of your work. As Howard Hodgkin put it, "Being an artist in England is like being in enemy territory."

The quest to find places where the grass is greener is a personal journey for most artists. It's a slow process of assessing existing contacts and interests, developing knowledge about the market for fine art, crafts or contemporary photography in different countries, networking with artists abroad and may well include pursuing individual inclinations and hunches.

However it would be wrong to jump from 'My work doesn't sell in Britain' to 'I must start exporting – it's bound to sell in America/Germany/Japan where people really appreciate art.' It is highly likely that if you can't sell your work in your own country you won't be able to sell it elsewhere. Why is this and what can you do about it?

If it is not selling here, you need to take a long hard look at what you are making and how you are marketing it. Successful marketing of any product, and art is no exception, involves a combination of four key elements:

• Product
• Place
• Price
• Promotion.

Is the work well made, original and interesting? Are you trying to sell it in inappropriate places? Have you researched thoroughly all the places where it could sell in your own locality, region and country? Have a look at the prices – perhaps they are too high or even too low. How well do you promote yourself? Good slides, a well-written CV, perhaps some postcards are a minimum in order to promote yourself at a distance.

Your move into exporting should be from a position of strength. It's all too easy to dismiss the real opportunities and creative freedom artists experience in Britain. Simone ten Hompel was born in Germany and did a traditional apprenticeship as a locksmith-blacksmith. Since coming to London to study at the RCA, she has settled here. She finds that Britain offers the freedom to do what she wants in her work. She particularly appreciates the experimentation-based approach to designer-made work in the UK and her innovative fine metalwork is widely praised. Simone occasionally sells work overseas but feels no need to actively pursue export markets.

If selling is your prime aim in developing an export market, you usually have to prove to overseas buyers that your work is a success on your home ground before they will take the risk of placing orders with you. You need to have developed a high level of confidence and professionalism from dealing with galleries and shops in this country before taking on different cultures and languages elsewhere. And it is likely that the success in this country is necessary to provide the resources for you to begin the slower, riskier and more expensive process of developing outlets overseas.

But once you have established a reputation and some selling success in the UK, starting to export is an excellent idea. It can improve your business success and ensure your survival as an artist or maker who can live from sales of your work.

Larger orders, better payment terms and greater selling opportunities can all come through exporting. Sally Penn-Smith who makes hand-painted glassware sells in Japan, the USA and Saudi

Arabia. She has found that "exporting is brilliant. In the UK orders are small and galleries often ask for sale or return. But export orders are much larger and are paid proforma, in advance of dispatch, direct into my bank account in sterling."

New horizons

What other benefits have artists and makers gained from exporting? Sometimes exporting can be a way of doing something you just cannot do in your own country. Perhaps UK artists are less driven by this than artists living in very small, isolated countries where cultural expression is limited. But both economic and aesthetic concerns can motivate artists to look elsewhere.

'Wearable art' is a more recognised phenomenon in the United States than in Britain and a number of galleries and shops offer textile artists in this field greater opportunities than on their home ground. Recession in the UK with a lack of investment in building projects inspired furniture designer-maker Nick Allen to look to Hong Kong for commissions through architects and design consultancies. Ceramicist Jenny Beavan finds that not many British galleries and collectors relate to her work. By promoting herself internationally in Germany and the Netherlands she has found far more people who understand and appreciate what she is doing.

Key points

- The decision to export can be motivated by many factors: desire for an international reputation, seeking to feel part of an international community of artists and for business survival.
- For many the initial decision to export is unplanned rather than planned.
- Don't invest a lot of effort in investigating export markets until you have explored the full potential for selling and exhibiting your work in the UK.
- Sometimes an artist needs to export in order to work in a way which is not possible in the UK, for economic or aesthetic reasons.

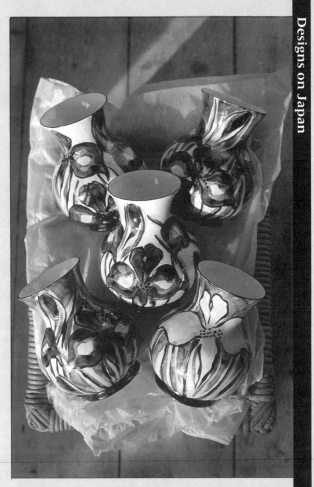

Annie Doherty,
**hand-painted fine
bone china**

Annie Doherty creates colourful exuberant designs for china tableware. She makes one-off handpainted pieces and is also successful in selling her designs. Marks and Spencer commissioned a range of designs from her and she is keen to work more in this way. In 1992 she was approached by a Japanese company proposing to market her designs in Japan.

After a lengthy period of negotiation, Annie is travelling to Japan in 1994 for two exhibitions of her work in Tokyo. The shows have been set up by the licensing company in partnership with the Circle Gallery. As is common in Japan, they take place in a department store and central shopping area of the Ginza where the gallery has a concession.

These shows will be used by the licensing company to launch Annie Doherty as a designer in Japan. As well as selling one-off pieces specially made for the exhibitions, the company will introduce her to ceramics, textile and stationery producers with a view to selling the designs. The company has commissioned a large quantity of work for the show, have organised shipping and are paying up front for the work and her travel expenses.

Annie acknowledges that she is a little nervous about the trip because doing business with the Japanese is so different. Her preparation includes useful advice on negotiating contracts from a cousin who works in Tokyo. She has discovered that prices are very much higher than in the UK but has been advised that strict rules are observed in Japan when negotiating a price. Never accept the first figure offered and have the confidence to propose a higher alternative is the basic principle.

She also recognises that speaking no Japanese and being dependent on the company who organise the visit will make doing business in Tokyo altogether different from operating on home ground.

With prior experience of licensing designs, she has requested a sample contract from the Japanese company and will get a UK solicitor to check it before her trip. An area of particular concern is whether designs are to be licensed for use in Japan only or for export. Annie knows how vital it is to ensure that cheaper exports do not compete with her individually handpainted work which sells well in galleries and shops in Britain and the USA.

She had to deal with one such problem when straight copies of her work made in the Philippines turned up in shops in Britain. Legal advice determined that she could not sue the manufacturing firm but had to take secondary action against the shops stocking the work. A solicitor's letter notifying them that she was about to take legal action against them resulted in an out of court settlement.

See page 26, 'Licensing reproductions' in 3 • The artist's experience

In reality, sueing the importers could have cost up to £15,000, a risk few makers would be able to take. So protecting your design copyright is essential. A contract to license a design should specify a one-off payment and royalties according to the number of times the design is used. Because of the difficulty of monitoring the use of her designs in Japan, Annie reckons it may be better to settle for a larger initial payment and smaller royalties. The reverse is usually the case in the UK.

3 • The artist's experience

Exporting is a business term which describes the process of selling your product to an overseas customer. Any publication on running a business will include advice on exporting. There might be sections on developing export markets, export intelligence, export credit guarantees, inward and outward trade missions. They tend to describe large overseas markets and often the language seems to belong to a world of espionage and military campaigns.

So it can be difficult for artists to relate this definition of exporting to what they make and their own reasons for wanting to work internationally. The 'product' which artists and craftspeople make is individual and unique. It is not designed to be exported to mass markets or show strongly in overseas trade statistics.

Artists therefore need to develop their own broader definition of exporting which places at the heart of the process artworks crossing borders. In some circumstances it also includes artists and materials crossing borders. With this broader definition, a number of different purposes can be identified, which form the basis for 'exporting' as explored in this book.

Selling work abroad

This is the most straightforward area of exporting and includes direct selling (eg at a market), receiving orders from an overseas gallery or shop and mail order. It may be a one-off experience as with a market or involve repeat orders. In both cases reliable methods of transportation and payment must be researched. The following examples illustrate this area of exporting.

London designer-makers in demand in Tokyo
Textile artists Emma Sewell and Harriet Wallace-Jones started trading as Wallace Sewell in 1992. Their fine woven scarves and other items were spotted at Chelsea Craft Fair by buyers for department stores

Jenny Beavan, **pair of teapots with stands,** *Rock Formation in Thin Section*, **porcelain, with river mud, coloured slips and locally found materials, 1993. Photo:** the artist

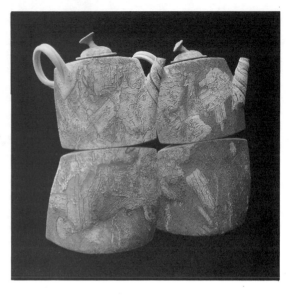

Since she was awarded membership of the International Academy of Ceramics, Jenny Beavan **has come into contact with many overseas ceramicists and this network has been the key to international opportunities. She won the Inax Design Award in 1989: the prize included a three month work and study visit to Japan. She has exhibited in Lebanon, the USA, Germany, Japan, Turkey, Holland and Belgium in the past six years. In 1993 she won the prestigious Vallauris ceramics biennial in France. She finds that reviews of such events reach collectors of fine ceramics internationally. An American buyer recently tracked her work down in Cornwall, having seen a review of a Netherlands exhibition in an American magazine. Jenny acknowledges that there is a paradox in her international success: she exhibits abroad because her work does not fit easily into ceramics traditions in this country. However, in showing abroad, she is seen as representing British ceramics in some way.**

in Japan and the USA. So, before they had established themselves in the UK, Wallace Sewell became involved in making large export orders. The stores provided detailed 'Vendor Instructions' but for the first-time exporter these are quite complex. Emma Sewell reckons it took them a year to really feel confident about exporting. They now have separate export price lists and are less daunted by the paperwork.

Finnish poster campaign

Rhonda Wilson is a photographer based in the West Midlands. Her work is based on social issues such as homelessness and low pay. Some commissions result in a series of images which are produced as a set of posters in a limited edition. Rhonda retains some to sell herself. A flyer inserted in *Creative Camera* magazine resulted in an order from a gallery in Finland. The posters were sent by mail and as a result Rhonda's work was part of an exhibition there on social documentary photography entitled 'Real Stories'. She was invited to speak at a gallery seminar and enjoyed a paid trip to Finland to attend the exhibition.

German ceramics market success

In August 1993 Clare and John Brelstaff travelled from their home in Cleveland with a carload of Clare's ceramics to the annual Oldenburg Töpfermarkt (Potter's Market) in Northern Germany. They had heard about the market through their daughter who was studying German there and helped them fill out the application form. John acknowledges they had little professional experience of selling work but they were delighted to take enough over the two day event to cover transport costs. They are keen to participate in other such events in Germany and France.

Exhibiting abroad

Exhibiting abroad involves artworks crossing borders and can be described as exporting for artists, whether or not the work is sold. In many countries customs procedure for sending work overseas for an exhibition will be different depending on whether work is for sale or not.

London paintings to Cologne – via Cadiz

Trisha Clarke is a painter based in London. She is involved in promoting her work in Europe through her company EuroArt. In November 1992 she organised a selection of work for a show at Arte Elemental in Cadiz in Southern Spain. Her unsold work from this exhibition was taken to a Cologne gallery for the annual Kunsttage (Art Day) gallery promotion and more sold. She hired a general removals carrier with a regular run to Spain to transport the work.

Clothes shows in New York and San Francisco

Carole Waller is a painter who makes clothes. She has found that there is a small network of galleries and shops in the USA which are interested in exhibiting and selling 'wearable art'. In 1992 she had one person shows at the Julie Gallery in New York and Obiko in San Francisco. In 1993 she took part in group exhibitions in galleries in Milwaukee and Boston. A number of shops in the USA stock her work. In the UK there are fewer opportunities for an artist working across the fine art/clothing boundary to exhibit in galleries. Carole uses UPS delivery services and has always found them extremely reliable. In the US import duty is payable by the person receiving the package. For clothing it is around 7%.

Trade fairs

Many makers and artists with experience of UK trade fairs turn to overseas events. At a trade only fair, samples are shown and these will usually be sold (or bartered with fellow exhibitors) at the end. Some fairs are open to the public in which case more stock must be taken. These fairs are most common in the decorative accessories, giftware, interiors, craft, jewellery and textiles fields and for many individual makers in the UK attendance has become a regular part of their year's activities. In the fine art field, groups of artists will occasionally take stands at overseas art fairs. However, it is more common for galleries to take stands, acting as agents for several artists.

Porcelain exhibitor in Frankfurt

Susan Mason is a ceramicist working in porcelain. She exhibited at the Frankfurt Handwerksmesse in 1992 and 1993 as part of a group selected through an East Midlands Arts initiative. The fair is the largest international event devoted to handmade craft products and attracts substantial numbers of buyers. Although she received no orders in 1992, Susan enjoyed considerable success on her second showing. She has supplied shops and galleries in Germany and elsewhere in Europe and hopes to build on this with a third visit to Frankfurt in 1994.

Liverpool designers take New York by storm

For the past six years textile design students at John Moores University have shown at the unique New York Surtex fair. On the broad theme of 'surface texture', exhibitors show a huge range of decorative products all concerned with pattern and design. Tutors at the University organise a stand through a DTI-subsidised scheme, take a range of work made by current students in textiles and fashion, and sell work with great success. Contacts have been made leading to placements for students with design studios in New York and elsewhere.

Hampshire glassmaker shows in Paris and Middle East

Jonathan Andersson works in glass and metal and is enthusiastic about the opportunities offered by trade and retail fairs overseas. In 1992 he showed at a large fair in Dubai. Subsidy from the DTI helped cover the costs, he sold all his samples but returned with no further orders. However, in the same year he went to the Paris Ateliers d'Art Show (PAAS), showing in the Ob'Art section which features quality one-off pieces. Here, apart from receiving a number of orders, he won an exhibitor's prize which covered the cost of the trip. Subsequently he had a solo exhibition in a French gallery with sales netting £12,000. In 1994 he plans to do the Paris show again and has been selected to show at an art fair in Miami, the largest of its kind in the USA with over 750,000 visitors in three days.

Open exhibitions and competitions

In theory this should be as straightforward as submitting an entry for an open event in the UK. In practice, an initial selection may be made from slides, but you often have to submit the actual work at an early stage. Great care must be taken to respect the regulations imposed by the event organisers, to ensure the security of the work submitted and to obtain its safe return. Open exhibitions and international competitions for artists and makers are advertised in *Artists Newsletter*, *Crafts* and fine art magazines. The comprehensive *Directory of International Open Art Exhibitions* gives submission details and prizes for competitions and open shows in 21 European countries.

See 13 • Further Reading

Cornish ceramicist wins Vallauris award

Jenny Beavan, a Cornwall-based ceramicist, entered the prestigious Vallauris International Ceramics Biennial in 1992 and won the AVOCA prize worth FF15000 (approximately £1750). After an initial selection from slide submissions, successful applicants were invited to send work for the exhibition. The regulations give precise instructions on packing and transport: for example, work must not be sent by parcel post. Prizes are only awarded when the jury views the exhibition. Regardless of value, all works awarded prizes in excess of FF10000 (approximately £1100) become the property of the Organisation Committee and join the collection of the International Museum of Ceramic Arts in Vallauris.

Overseas commissions

Many artists and makers are interested in doing work to commission. But undertaking commissions for overseas clients, while an attractive proposition, is complex and needs careful management. It is a good idea to develop such exporting opportunities through an experienced agent (for example, a gallery or design consultancy) who can liaise with the client. Many artists find that other countries offer greater

Vivienne Baker, *Breakfast in Portugal*, **oil on canvas, 1m x 1m, 1993**

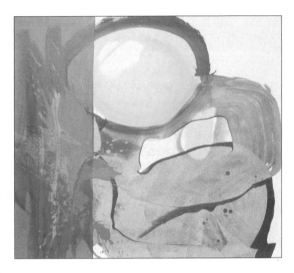

Vivienne Baker **was one of four artists from Bristol's Artspace Studios who spent four weeks in Oporto in 1993 as part of a studio exchange. They worked in a beautiful house belonging to the Taylors Port company, offered through a connection with the Bristol-Oporto society (the two cities are twinned).**

Apart from some communication problems before they set out, the exchange went very smoothly and was an intense and productive period of work for the four artists. Three worked in 3-D and donated their work to Taylors. Vivienne's work was more portable but could not return with her as it was on exhibition in Oporto. It eventually found its way back to Bristol via a Portuguese artist (friend of a friend) who was attending Shave Artists' Workshop in Somerset – an inexpensive solution to a practical problem using artists' networks.

opportunities to undertake commissions. With the right approach, this can become an exciting and satisfying area of work as the following examples show.

UK artist opens doors in Hong Kong

Nick Allen, an artist-designer working in wood, metal and glass has undertaken four commissions in Hong Kong over 18 months in 1992-93. The first, developed through an agent in London, was for an imposing entrance door with etched glass panels. This was made for a private client who initially wanted to look at furniture and purchase some door handles. When Nick realised the client had no door to put the handles on he proposed a more radical design approach and won a substantial commission. Nick has had to learn quickly the very different culture of doing business in Hong Kong.

Painting for Portuguese client

Lucinda Denning's large colourful painting in a Covent Garden gallery attracted the attention of a Portuguese business visitor to London. Unfortunately for the client, by the time he returned to the gallery, the painting had become part of *The Guardian*'s Art for Sale event where it immediately sold to another buyer. However, gallery owner Susie Fisher persuaded the client to commission a new work. A contract was agreed for a commission totalling £2800. For an initial fee

Lucinda is painting a series of cartoons from which the final work will be selected.

Transportation

See page 71, 'Other barriers to trade' in 8 • Getting it there

When artists are invited to undertake residencies and workshops in other countries and need specific materials, unobtainable in that country, for their work, they may decide to take their own. Artists travelling to another country to develop their work with the inspiration of a different environment, either on a painting holiday or by renting temporary studio accommodation elsewhere, may do the same.

If you know that local sources are expensive or unreliable in quality or supply, you will want to take a range of materials and equipment. However, be warned that carrying large quantities (eg for a workshop) may be viewed as a form of trade and incur import duty.

You should also be aware that some art materials in common use contravene regulations on the carriage of dangerous goods. In this case they are considered to be a safety hazard in transportation and are banned on aircraft. No item with a flash point under 60.5° Celsius can be carried on an airplane and certain oil colour mediums and varnishes fall into this category. You are advised to get a list from the manufacturers of any product you are carrying, stating the flashpoint of the product. A phone call to the airline is a good idea to ensure that providing information from manufacturers will allow you to transport your art materials.

Oil paints banned by airline

Painter Ted Schofield wrote to *Artists Newsletter* in 1993 describing how he discovered the hard way that it is illegal to carry certain oil paints in hand luggage on aircraft. The paints were confiscated when his luggage was checked at Gatwick although he was able to collect them when he returned to the country.

And occasionally, the sort of materials used by artists can arouse the interest of Customs Officers who view them as something else altogether.

Sculptor blocked from importing animal feed

Gligor Stafanov, an environmental sculptor based in the UK, was invited to Dublin in 1991 to create a work for the European City of Culture. Gligor works with natural materials and planned to take these with him including a quantity of straw. However the Customs Officers had other ideas. They declared the straw to be an illegal import of 'living animal feed' and impounded it.

Moving studio

Some artists and makers decide to relocate in another country as a permanent move. In this case the transporting of household goods, equipment, materials and finished work will be a major event. It is likely that the activity will be deemed to be 'importing' by the receiving country and import taxes or VAT may be incurred. If at some stage you plan to return to the UK, it is a good idea to keep full documentation of goods transported, otherwise you can become liable for import duties in both directions.

Licensing reproductions

Selling copyright licences so that reproductions of your work or your designs are marketed abroad is an entirely different area of exporting. Clearly you will not be involved in transporting artworks across borders and it may be possible to deal with the business aspects in this country.

See 13 • Further reading

This is a specialised area and artists should refer to AN Publications Artists Handbook on *Copyright* and the Visual Artists Contract for *Licensing Reproductions*. If you already have some experience of licensing use of your work in this country, you will be familiar with the issues and terminology. Dealing with overseas markets raises other issues such as whether the reproduction or design will be exported to the UK. Think carefully about this as it might be detrimental to sales of your original works.

Key points

- Artists' experience of exporting is varied and offers a huge range of interesting opportunities.
- Artists and makers need to define their own international focus, which may not necessarily involve selling work.
- Working internationally has led many artists to find overseas buyers and galleries keen to purchase and show their work.

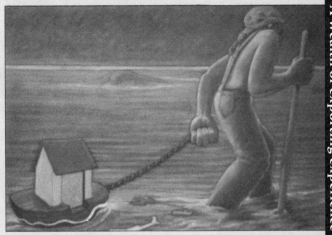

Mark
Goldsworthy,
Departure, **36"x
48", oil on
canvas, 1991.
Photo:** the artist

Artist Mark Goldsworthy has built up a range of experience exporting to several countries in different ways.

Firstly in 1989 and 1990 he exhibited small pictures with a gallery in Dinard in France but describes this as "a very uneasy relationship". He found that the owners fell back on proven 'sellers' and local artists and whenever any differences of opinion occurred they found "an inability to understand my French or enough English to communicate". This helped achieve a lack of that trust which is "essential when leaving your work in the hands of a stranger" and the low level of income from sales barely covered the expense of numerous trips to France.

In 1991 Mark found an exhibition space in Valenciennes, also in France. He took a show of his work over, hung it and returned a month later to collect the work. Local papers gave the exhibition some publicity but Mark found it difficult to advertise the show properly since he did not have an appropriate mailing list for the region. Sales were low and the costs of transporting work to France and back were quite high but he did enjoy the experience of retaining control over the selection and presentation of the work and organising the space.

Around this time, Mark was involved in a mixed show which was part of a cultural exchange between the twin towns of Norwich and Rouen. Selected artists submitted two works, there was no cost to the artist and the show was in a contemporary gallery in Rouen. However he did not hear of any work selling. The exhibition seemed to be more about using the artists' work to promote the city abroad, the artists being pushed to the background.

Then in 1993, as part of a group of eight artists, he had an exchange exhibition with artists from Norway. The Norwegian artists exhibited at The Contact Gallery in Norwich. Mark and others took the work to Norway and returned three weeks later to collect the show. Each artist contributed £150 towards costs. Sales were slow but the artists who visited Norway were "treated admirably and enjoyed themselves". They agreed it was a very worthwhile show although Mark recognises that inexperience caused some delays at Customs. Before the exhibition, the artists contacted the DTI who informed them they should raise a Carnet, costing £100. They were also advised that if the total value of work exceeded around £3,000, they would have to pay VAT on entering Norway which would be refunded when the work left the country. They got around this by pricing work low.

Also in 1993 he showed in a gallery in Vienna through a mixed show organised by Wilde Contemporary Art. Here there was a fee of £250 to participating artists and a reduced commission of 20% on work sold. Having exhibited with the gallery in London before, Mark was left to make his own selection of paintings, "a freedom that I have not experienced elsewhere", and showed six good-sized pictures, thus creating an exhibition within an exhibition which gave a strong representation of his work. He gave the gallery permission to negotiate from the asking price, a fact which he feels secured the sale of a large oil painting to an art collector, with the promise of future sales.

From all these experiences, Mark Goldsworthy describes the four things he has found important to success:

- To be able to trust the people you are dealing with and for them to be able to trust you to provide a show that is professional.

- It is helpful if one person, not the artist, is responsible for publicity and drawing up a mailing list.

- When you spend money in participating in an overseas exhibition, expect the worst, ie no sales. Try to allow a certain amount of flexibility in every direction.

- Include in the prices an allowance for any unexpected expenses.

4 • Planning & preparation

Planning and preparation are the key to successful exporting. Remember that dealing with galleries, shops, commissioning bodies and agents at a distance can be more complicated and risky than working close to home. Chasing up any problems that may occur will involve you in far greater expense and time than in dealing with the same situation in your own country. Prepare yourself by answering some crucial questions before you start.

- Am I ready to export?
- Where can I get advice and information from?
- Are there any grants available to help me export?
- Which countries should I target?
- How do I find the right galleries and shops there?
- Do I need to be able to speak the language?

Ready to export?

This is a really basic question. All the advice from experts points one way. You need to be sure you have explored (and exploited) the potential for selling in your own country before you even think about exporting. As Sean O'Farrell, Development Officer at the Crafts Council of Ireland, points out: "Mistakes are cheaper at home. It's a less painful, less expensive training ground."

Being ready to export is all about professionalism, confidence and competence. Can you present yourself and your work professionally? If you already have some experience of selling and exhibiting in your own country, the chances are you can. Negotiation skills, essential for survival as a self-employed artist, will be vital for dealing with overseas buyers. Can you negotiate with confidence? And what about the business side? It's certainly not as straightforward as selling in your own country so you need a good level of competence to deal with it. If you pack the wrong delivery note when sending work to a UK gallery, it's not likely to be too disastrous. A couple of phone calls can sort it out. But getting export documentation wrong can be costly and time-consuming. At worst, you may end up having to pay to receive returned goods which couldn't be delivered because of errors in the paperwork. And if it's packed badly and not insured, you might lose it altogether – and lose a customer as well.

So getting ready to export means assessing your own levels of competence, confidence and professionalism. However, there may be some short cuts or intermediary stages to exporting which are worth exploring first. UK trade fairs, appropriate for most makers and some fine artists, are a good way of reaching overseas buyers who place export orders. Export buying houses or merchandising houses based in the UK represent overseas businesses who purchase work direct.

There are many other ways of bringing your work to the attention of overseas buyers while staying at home. The UK is well-placed for this with a number of major trade fairs, buying houses, shops and galleries attracting international buyers from Europe, the USA, Japan and the Middle East.

Sometimes it's right to ignore advice

In spite of all this good advice, some artists without extensive home-based experience are ready to export. Sheer determination, energy and curiosity, often combined with strategic contacts in other countries, give them the will to succeed.

When an artist's vision of working internationally comes from a desire to relate to artists and their work in other countries, rather than from pure business survival, they are likely to get involved in working overseas without ever calling it exporting. Such a vision can be a strong motivation and if pursued single-mindedly is likely to lead to success.

Advice, information & grants

So you know you want to export. What's the next step?

There are a large number of agencies and organisations who carry information on exporting, which is good news for artists and makers. But the bad news is it can be difficult to find out exactly what they all do. Changes instituted by central government and regional variations mean that the names and responsibilities of these agencies may vary in different parts of the country.

The way many of the agencies aim to help you is by 'signposting' which means they direct you to others who are more suited to your needs. This is not necessarily all that helpful. In practice it can mean that you ring agency A who tell you to contact agencies B and C. Ring agency B and they will tell you to contact agencies A and C. By the time you ring agency C you have a good idea what they will suggest you do. It can be a frustrating process since staff come over as highly trained in the art of passing you on rather than listening to and answering your questions. An article in *The Guardian* in 1993 described how the "present structure of support and advice for smaller firms is so fragmented that businesses are put off by the 'bewilderment factor'. There are so many competing and conflicting sources that they do not know where to go."

However, a new solution is planned which involves the setting up of One-Stop Shops. A number have been piloted in 1993 and it is aimed to establish these across the country in the next few years. The idea is to offer a single source of information for businesses and exporting is one of the areas to be covered. The One-Stop Shops are targeting small and medium-sized businesses.

It can also be difficult for artists and makers who want to start exporting to know what questions to ask. None of the agencies like to be asked vague questions such as 'I am an artist and I want to export to America. What should I do?' So there's a process of getting hold of all the relevant free literature, drawing up your own checklist of questions, making them as precise as possible and directing them to the right agency.

The principle UK agencies providing advice and information on exporting are listed below. Some also provide grants to help with the initial expenses involved in exporting.

Department of Trade and Industry (DTI)

The DTI is the UK government department dealing with all aspects of trade. It has offices in Scotland, Wales and Northern Ireland and eight regional offices in England. The Overseas Trade Services network provides practical help, advice and support to UK exporters. They produce a large number of publications and can help with consultancy in export marketing, market research and a whole range of other services.

The main priority for the DTI will always be larger companies so it can be hard for artists and makers to find what they need from them. But with some imagination and persistence, the DTI can be extremely useful. Anyone considering exporting should ring their DTI National or Regional Office and obtain the free booklets which give general advice: *Exporting: Guide to Exporting Services, UK Export Information Services, Specific Export Help* and *Overseas Promotion.* Other free booklets target specific markets, eg *Trading within Europe.*

You have to pay for other specialised reports. The *Hints to Exporters* series and *Country Profiles,* costing from £5-15, are available for a large number of countries. Comprehensive market reports, costing around £30, are available on specific sectors, for example 'How to Approach the Crafts Market' (USA), 'Interiors' (Japan) and 'Giftware' (New Zealand).

These and a huge array of market research information can be consulted at the DTI's Export Market Information Centre in London. The Crafts Council's library carries the relevant reports, as do most good business libraries and Chambers of Commerce. Always check for access as some libraries may be restricted to members' use only.

The DTI offers subsidy to businesses taking stands at designated overseas trade fairs. This is usually 50% of the stand costs and a contribution towards travel expenses. Selection for these fairs is through a 'joint venture sponsor'. The Overseas Promotion section of the DTI can provide a list of trade fairs with their joint venture sponsors. For example, the Crafts Council selects UK participants for the New York Gift Fair, the British Knitting and Clothing Export Council select makers of all types of gifts and accessories for most of the overseas fashion and design fairs.

Specific questions on particular countries can be answered by ringing the relevant DTI Country Desk. These telephone numbers are available from the DTI and are listed in their free booklets under 'Market Branches'.

Another useful service offered by the DTI is 'New Products from Britain' where for a small fee they will write, translate and place an article on your product in the relevant trade press of any country you choose. This scheme has been used very effectively by a number of craftspeople. Of course your work needs to be suitable to be considered for this service: the keywords are 'product' and 'trade press' so it's probably not appropriate for most fine artists.

Training and Enterprise Councils (TECs)
Also known as Local Enterprise Councils (LECs) in Scotland, the TECs were set up by the Department of Employment with a broad brief to provide business advice and counselling, consultancy and training for small businesses. They are all run independently and offer different ranges of services such as the government support scheme

Esther Ward, *Neckpiece*,
**stainless steel, paper and PVA
glue, 1992. Photo:** F.X.P.
Photography

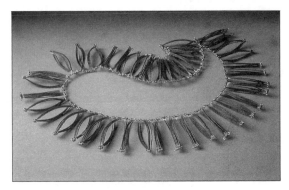

**Esther Ward exhibits and sells
her stainless steel jewellery in
the USA, Germany and the
Netherlands.** She has never
actively promoted her work
abroad but international
opportunities have developed
from showing work at the
prestigious Galerie Ra in
Amsterdam and Electrum in
London. She currently sells
well in America through an
agent who, through his own
Dutch connections, saw her
work in Galerie Ra. This agent
actively promotes Esther's
work by taking it around
galleries and putting together
themed exhibitions. He has
even sold work to public
collections in the States.
Initially the agent worked for
an annual fee but has now
moved onto a mark-up basis
only. Esther finds sending
work by post is easiest but
she's aware it offers
inadequate insurance cover
for her purposes. However,
others in the business are just
as trusting in their approach:
she once received a parcel
from Germany containing
£500 in cash labelled
'Photographic materials'!

to small businesses where a business adviser can offer you up to three free counselling sessions at your place of work.

You may also come into contact with your TEC through the Enterprise Allowance Scheme (operating under different names around the country). Ask what advice they can provide and request any free publications on exporting such as the Department of Employment's *How to Start Exporting*.

One-Stop Shops

These are in the process of being set up across the country having been piloted in 1993 in Birmingham, Cheshire, Hertfordshire, Manchester and Tyneside. One-Stop Shops should provide library and information services on a range of business issues including exporting and marketing. However it seems unlikely that they will become the single source of information since there are no plans to close down other existing agencies. But One-Stop Shops should be useful as the obvious starting point for small businesses and self-employed artists seeking business information.

Banks

Many banks have small business advisers and produce literature on a range of issues including exporting. Contact your local branch for details.

Euro Info Centres (EIC)

There are 21 EICs in the UK, set up by the European Commission to help small and medium-sized companies develop business in Europe. EICs offer a range of information on exporting in Europe, including identifying business partners in other countries, regulations concerning standards, packaging and labelling and some provide translation services. Charges for their services are fixed by each centre although you should be able to get an initial short consultation free of charge. If you want to export to Europe, contact your local EIC to see what they can offer – the service varies greatly across the country.

Chambers of Commerce

These are independently-run organisations, with a membership fee, which offer different services around the country. Chambers of Commerce are the outlet for the DTI's Active Exporting Scheme. This offers a specialist advice for small businesses from an Export Development Advisor to determine how you could benefit from exporting and how to plan for export success. This may involve an initial free 'export audit' followed by a fee-paying consultancy. Other services offered by Chambers of Commerce include export documentation, market research, library services, advice on regulations and payments.

The most comprehensive range of services is generally offered by those Chambers of Commerce located in major cities. Some services are for members only but DTI export development schemes, the issuing of Carnets and other export documentation services are available to all. Most major Chambers of Commerce will deal with brief specific telephone enquiries about exporting from non-members.

Customs and Excise

Customs and Excise are responsible for collecting VAT and can provide official guidelines on export documentation. While few artists are registered for VAT (the annual turnover for registration in 1994 is £45,000), VAT can affect artists who sell abroad and is described in '9 • Sales administration'.

Any VAT registered trader who requires specific advice on importing or exporting should send their enquiry in writing to Customs & Excise prior to undertaking the transaction and describe exactly what they propose doing. Under the terms of their guidelines, Customs & Excise should respond within ten days and give you written instruction on what to do. As long as this advice is followed, it is almost impossible for Customs then to impose a penalty.

Artists and makers involved in exporting should always refer to Customs & Excise documentation and advice services for the latest information. Guidelines and legislation do change quite frequently. VAT traders in particular should take great care as the penalties for errors can be high. Customs have no sympathy with mistakes because the advice service is available.

Debra O'Mahoney (Etoile Design), Embroidered gold star on irridescent velvet

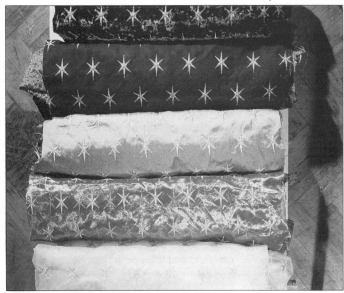

Debra designs and makes embroidery, working with some of the top fashion designers in the world. Export sales have grown with the business, which she set up in 1991. She received useful guidance from the Export Development Adviser at the London Chamber of Commerce, arranged through the Prince's Youth Business Trust. She visits trade shows, goes twice a year to France and Italy, has an Italian agent and is increasing her export sales. Distance is no problem. She works for clients in New York, discussing the design brief on the phone, then faxing through some designs and once approved, they send her the fabric to embroider. Debra attributes her success to having "an open mind and lots of common sense" and "not being afraid to jump on a plane or cold call a fashion company in Italy, even when I don't speak Italian!"

Arts funding bodies

All these organisations run specialist programmes of support and are likely to be more oriented towards working internationally as a way of developing creatively rather than pure exporting.

They may organise training on, for example, 'Marketing in Europe' and provide travel bursaries or financial assistance with trade fairs. East Midlands Arts ran a specialist seminar for craftspeople in 1993 called 'Trading Places' on promoting crafts in Europe with gallery owners from France, Germany and the Netherlands. Some arts funding bodies organise regular international exchanges, eg South East Wales Arts Association exchanges with Philadelphia and Rajasthan; the Scottish Arts Council has studio residencies in Australia and Amsterdam. The Visual Arts Officer at your regional arts board may be able to put you in touch with another artist who is exhibiting or selling in a particular country.

The Crafts Council runs the Picture Bank, Europe's first publicly accessible electronic picture library which is consulted by international buyers and visitors. The library carries many international craft magazines. The Council can provide information on international publications, competitions and galleries and is preparing a series of international fact sheets.

Local authority economic development units

Local authorities have a concern with the healthy economic development of their area. There is generally a section in the council with special responsibility for business development. Find out whether they offer any information or programme of support for small businesses which want to export. Some councils offer grants for 'marketing missions' to other European countries, assisting with travel costs to enable you to visit shops, galleries or attend a trade fair in order to sell your work.

Business initiatives for younger artists

Specialist advice is available from two agencies: Livewire, for 16-25s, and for under 30s the Prince's Youth Business Trust (PYBT). Advisers can help you draw up a business plan, devise a marketing strategy and plan for exporting.

Livewire have set up a new scheme called 'Export Challenge' which will give young owner-managers specialist export training and advice. A trade mission to mainland Europe is planned.

PYBT offers selected businesses subsidised stands at high-profile trade fairs where you are likely to encounter international buyers. Every year 200 nominated businesses exhibit at the PYBT showcase during the Autumn Gift Fair (a huge international trade fair) in Birmingham's NEC. Research shows that 20-30% of orders taken there are for export. PYBT are negotiating a special package for their selected businesses to obtain export development advice from the Chamber of Commerce.

Artists Newsletter

The newsletter carries an international section, listing opportunities such as open exhibitions abroad, residencies and competitions.

Targeting the right place

The DTI and other bodies can provide statistics for a country's economic production, levels of imports, consumer spending in particular sectors. However as art is not a standard 'product' these may not be that helpful. When you start exporting, you'll need to look at other factors.

Firstly, since art and fine craft are never essential purchases, you need to identify countries with a reasonably healthy economic environment. Statistics can help. Asking someone who has travelled there recently put you in the picture in a more direct way.

Open to innovation

The other important area to assess is how open people are to things that are new, different and come from elsewhere. In general a multi-cultural, well-educated and well-travelled population will be most open to innovative work. Such people are often to be found in the major cities and certain tourist areas. Isolated countries with well-defined cultural identities and their own strong design aesthetic may be more closed to work from other places. But the same is not true of Japan, a country which maintains its own strong cultural identity while exercising a huge appetite for all things new. So look carefully and start to home in on cities and regions rather than whole countries.

Magazine culture

Your research should be combined with a close study of any art, design, craft, style and interiors magazines from that particular country you can lay your hands on. The Crafts Council, National Art Library at the Victoria and Albert Museum and national cultural institutes such as the French Institute and the Goethe Institut have libraries (check for hours and public access).

Specialist art, craft and photography journals will give you gallery listings and shops. They will tell you how much work is exhibited from other countries. They'll give you a feel for what work is critically appreciated.

More general magazines carry important clues on style, fashion, level of visual awareness. In most cases, just looking at the advertisements will give you an idea of the level of visual sophistication and design awareness. Do you like what you see? Try to imagine your work in the context the magazines present – would it look extraordinarily colourful and flamboyant, or rather subtle? Do any humorous or political references translate into another culture? For example, work dealing with environmental issues might be understood and appreciated in the Netherlands or California but less so in Southern Europe.

All this will help you identify your own starting points. The next stage is committing yourself to a particular market and planning a more detailed strategy.

Speaking the language

If you want to develop a long-term business connection with another country, speaking the language is always going to be an advantage. But don't forget that English is widely spoken. In the Netherlands, Scandinavia and the German-speaking countries, you won't have too many problems but in France, Spain and Italy you're less likely to encounter fluent English speakers. Many international buyers from the Middle and Far East are used to dealing with the USA and will speak English. However, it is always a courtesy to learn some basic words in the language of the country and one which is much appreciated.

What can be more important in the initial stages is to develop an awareness of the country's culture, in how people relate to each other and do business. There are many books to help you. Guidance on, for example, how formal or informal you are expected to be, punctuality, negotiation practice, whether business decisions are made in the office or in a café can all help prepare you for a marketing trip. British people are often less well-travelled than their counterparts in mainland Europe and can come over as inflexible or ignorant in their attitudes. By understanding and accepting other ways of doing things, you will find you are more easily welcomed as a person to do business with.

Key points

- Assess whether you are ready to export and whether you have the professionalism, confidence and competence to deal with what can be a risky and expensive way of doing business.
- There are a lot of business and other agencies offering advice, information and some grants to help you get involved in exporting. Spend time gathering information and assessing what your own needs are.
- Identifying which countries to target is a first step. The next stage is vital: deciding which cities or regions to target and finding out where the galleries and shops are.
- Speaking the language of the country is important, even if it is only a few phrases. Learning about the culture and the way people do business is just as essential.

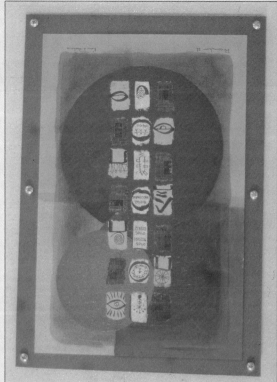

Ken Devine, *11 December 1993*, **420 x 295mm, print, acrylic & ink, 1993. Photo:** the artist

On December 11th 1993 at 19.00 hours Greenwich Mean Time seven exhibitions opened simultaneously in Portsmouth, Århus, Duisburg, Reykavik, Amsterdam, Moscow and Bratislava. Each featured work by the same 49 artists from the UK, Denmark, Germany, Iceland, Netherlands, Russia and Slovakia.

Artist Ken Devine formed the idea of the event, entitled '777 Distance Communication', following the 1992 'Europe in Portsmouth' festival. This brought together artists from across Europe and a special bond was made with artists from Russia and Slovakia.

The 777 feat of co-ordination involved networking internationally to contact seven artists or artists' groups in seven different countries. Each chose seven artists to participate in the network. Central to the project was that it remained artist-led, aiming "to enable visual artists in a broad European context to make work and exhibit it throughout the wider community whilst maintaining a high degree of control over what is and how it is communicated."

Each artist made seven pieces of work inspired by the theme 'Seven years to the Millennium'. The project determined that work should fit into an A3 package and be sent by post so that costs for each centre were not prohibitive. Each group also had to identify an exhibition space and negotiate the conditions and funding necessary to have an exhibition. The inauguration date was fixed when there was a positive commitment from all seven partners.

The works in sets of seven (one by each artist) were posted out to the participating galleries. Even though post was chosen as an easy form of transport, problems did occur. Work from Reykavik was impounded in London as it did not have a Carnet. It had to be returned to Iceland to get the relevant export documentation before being dispatched back to the UK. Work from the UK left for Bratislava without a Carnet – again on bad advice from the postal authorities – and was "stuck somewhere" a week before the exhibition opened.

Ken Devine describes the experience as "a very steep learning curve". He found that a year's lead-in time was not sufficient. The project's timing was inappropriate for some participants whose cycles for funding applications are different from the UK. But, by holding onto the original vision and having clear priorities, the 777 exhibition at Aspex Gallery in Portsmouth has been the start of an important new network of artists in Europe.

In the catalogue, produced in Portsmouth in the seven languages of the participating countries, Sandy Nairne emphasizes the networking principle. "777 follows the best current pattern of European development: de-centred and created out of strong links between equal partners." And Ken Devine underlines that "the ethos of the network has placed great emphasis on authorship and editorial control remaining in the place of origin" and "the whole project has relied on trust between individuals and respect for the decisions they have made. Through this process there is an inevitable diversity and it is this which 777 pursues absolutely."

Future plans include holding an artists' conference in 1994. The aim is to create a growing network of artists across Europe who want to organise their own exhibitions in other countries. Networking offers the appropriate means of communication for artists to share contacts and develop partnerships in order to achieve their objectives.

5 • Networking

Networking has become something of a buzzword in recent years. But it is something which has always come naturally to artists. Networking is quite simply a process of talking to other artists and sharing information. It involves recognising that in such an isolated profession there is a strong need to relate to each other, and that artists' interests can be best served by pooling ideas, resources and contacts.

Artists Newsletter performs a vital function in networking among artists. It provides a forum, whether on the letters page or in the opportunities section, for artists to inform each other, request help and contacts, raise questions for debate. Networking already happens naturally, in your own location, in your studio group, in specialist associations such as potters' and textile artists' groups. Contacting others via *Artists Newsletter* and specialist newsletters can be a way of widening your own network to include people you wouldn't otherwise meet.

What is essential about networking is that it comes out of a need to communicate regularly and involves relating to others as equals. It means giving as well as receiving. Some networks have become formalised into associations, membership organisations, specialist groups. But whether constituted, publicly funded, structured or informal, the principle of equality is fundamental to a network. And what you put in determines what you get out.

International networking

So how can networking help artists get involved in working internationally, in exporting their work, skills and ideas? Firstly, networking offers an array of possibilities of communicating with artists internationally. It doesn't just mean direct face-to-face contact.

Susan Derges, *The observer and the observed,* **black and white photograph, 36" x 48", 1991**

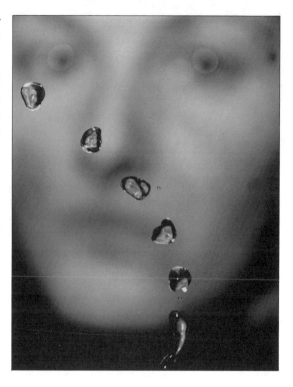

This image was part of a 1994 exhibition of Susan Derges' **work at James Danziger Gallery in New York. Susan's main experience of exhibiting overseas has come though living abroad and making contacts with artists. She lived in Japan for five years in the 1980s, researching audio-visual media and working. She had several exhibitions in Tokyo galleries, museums and department stores. In the 1970s she spent a year in Berlin on a DAAD scholarship. Her work is in the collections of Kunstlerhaus Bethanien and Neuer Berliner Kunstverein in Berlin and the Hara Museum in Tokyo. Susan's experience is that: "90% of things happen through artists. I've found that the way you start to make contact with artists in other countries is through relating to common issues in the work. Networking between artists is vital and can lead to many varied and interesting overseas opportunities."**

It can involve communication by post, phone, fax, electronic bulletin boards, newsletters, magazines and even mail art.

Mail art is really networking in a nutshell, an original solution to the desire among artists to communicate internationally. There's a principle of equality, it's inexpensive and involves a degree of trust among a community of like-minded individuals. Work on a determined theme, to a specified size, is sent to an unknown person in another country and exhibited there in return for 'full documentation' which can mean anything from a catalogue to a photocopied sheet of contributors. As Deedla Ludwig pointed out in *Artists Newsletter,* mail art started in the 1950s and has developed into a popular way of guaranteeing open access to mail art networks. Fluxus artist, Robert Filliou, named it the Eternal Network. Artist Royston Du Maurier-Lebek describes his experience: "Since 1991 I have sent off to every mail art request in *Artists Newsletter* and have had work shown in Russia, France, in fact the whole of Europe including the old communist states, the Americas north and south. It is a medium of getting your work, views and voice heard."

Networking through organisations

How else can artists develop international networking in order to achieve their objectives? There are a number of international organisations which offer scope for valuable networking. They may be open to membership by individual artists, such as the European Textile Network; be formed through a selection process of nominations, eg the International Academy of Ceramicists; act as an umbrella group representing the interests of existing organisations, eg the International Association of Art and the World Crafts Council-Europe. Many produce publications which share information among members on exhibition opportunities, funding and competitions.

Formal and informal networks can be a way of identifying individuals or groups who share your interests. It can be a way of developing joint projects or sharing information. In recent years British potters have participated in high quality potters' markets in the Netherlands and Germany. Initially the invitation to Josie Walter and a number of other potters came through their being featured in the Craft Potters Association's handbook, ie through networking. Now the markets have become more widely known and many are open to individual applications from UK potters. There is an interest in setting up a potters' market in this country. This could involve inviting some of the Dutch, Belgian and German potters who regularly attend these markets and have formed an informal network of participants.

Studio networking

Studio group exchanges are an excellent example of international networking among artists. In Bristol, Artspace studios has developed a relationship with studio groups in the city's twin towns of Bordeaux, Belfast, Hannover and Oporto. A number of exchanges have resulted with artists swapping both studio and home for four weeks. Exhibitions and commissions have also evolved through the relationships which have developed. In an *Artists Newsletter* article on international exchanges, Michelle Farmer, Artspace administrator, underlines the need for artists to confront the difference between cultures: "The last

Trevor Atkinson, *Rain Falling*, oil 20" x 30".

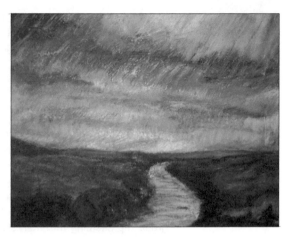

Trevor Atkinson **pursued all available artist contacts in the United States for two years, in an effort to set up an exchange exhibition, before receiving his first reply. Eventually someone there forwarded his request to an American sculpture magazine who published it in their listings section. Two artists replied, one in Minnesota and one in New Jersey, both inviting him to stay. On his first trip to the States, Trevor made many useful contacts. A second trip to New Jersey followed when, through his artist friends, he arranged to run workshops in schools and had an exhibition. Workshop fees and sales of work paid for the trip and he is planning a third visit. Trevor states: "My contact with American artists has completely changed my attitude. They are very professional and have an entirely different approach to selling and exhibiting. They have the confidence to charge high prices and know the value of their work. I have learned a lot from them and it has changed the way I work here."**

thing we want is for artists to simply continue the work they do, in a foreign town. We want people to be inspired by the place. We try and send people with different artistic outlooks. For instance, in Bordeaux we were working with a group of printmakers, so we sent abstract artists to see what they would make of it."

In Norwich, artists in St Ethelreda's studios developed an exchange partnership with artists in Estonia. Two artists travelled to Tallinn and funds were raised to enable six Estonian artists to spend time working in studios in Norwich and a joint exhibition resulted.

Networking starts at college

International networking is fostered by many art colleges. If your college is a member of ELIA (the European League of Institutes for the Arts), at least one member of staff will be involved in information exchange with a large number of art colleges across Europe. This network aims specifically to 'promote international cooperation between students and teachers of academic institutes of art throughout Europe' and to 'collect and disseminate information to establish/improve exchange programmes and joint projects'. The network should be a good starting point for contacting art students elsewhere.

Many colleges have established exchanges through ERASMUS or TEMPUS programmes where students spend a period of their studies in another art institute elsewhere in Europe.

Germinations Europe is a network which brings young artists together to practice and exhibit at an international level. Each year a small number of students and recent graduates under 30 are selected for a programme which in 1994 involved one-month workshops in Delphi, Breda, Bratislava or Liverpool, followed by an exhibition in the Netherlands. The process of participation creates its own networks. Contacts are built up with other participants and locally where the workshop takes place. Over a period of years, such contacts can lead to other exhibitions and opportunities.

In some ways networking works best within a group of people. Everyone gains substantially from the shared information and contacts and the competitive edge is dulled. But networking can be a good approach between two individuals. Trading information on, say, exhibition opportunities, shops and galleries, exchanging slides and CVs to get feedback from an artist in another country on your work and how you present yourself, might be valuable steps to establishing your reputation in that country – and their reputation here.

But remember, what you put in determines what you get out. Natural networkers communicate freely in order to achieve shared objectives. It's what you do with that information that counts.

Key points

- Networking is a vital process which can help artists to communicate internationally.
- The means of communication can take many forms.
- Networking grows out of a shared need to communicate on common issues. It is a two-way process involving giving as well as receiving.
- Artists can join formal networks such as international associations or develop their own informal networks through contacts made in a wide variety of ways.

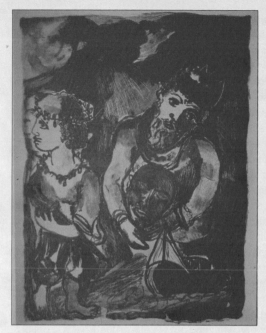

Juliette Goddard, *From the mouth of the volcano*, **stone lithograph.** **Photo:** the artist

Painter Juliette Goddard and ceramics artist Adam Sutherland have developed a reputation in Switzerland over the past seven years. It began with a family connection.

"We started by bringing over some paintings, prints and ceramics whenever we came on holiday to visit Adam's brother and took them round the galleries," explains Juliette. It was relatively easy to find their way around since Switzerland is a small country with a good number of galleries, both in medium-sized towns and in the cities. The main galleries are in Basel, due to the Art Fair, but Zürich is another major centre. The response was very encouraging: "Some galleries even bought work on the spot which is unheard of in England."

Over the years they worked to develop these contacts and gained the interest of galleries, collectors and commissioners. Juliette finds the Swiss appreciate original works such as oil paintings but prints are harder to sell. She reckons that she and Adam succeed because their work shows well against that of Swiss artists due to the figurative nature of their work. Much of modern Swiss art is abstract or minimalist, as well as very expensive.

Although Switzerland has the image of a traditional country with conservative tastes, she finds it to be very forward-looking and both older and younger people are keen to invest in contemporary work: "People love art in Switzerland. Many of the big employers have developed large collections that are housed in the work place." Juliette also finds buyers have a real interest in the artist. She was invited to the house of a purchaser of one of her paintings and requested to sign the 'Artists' Book'.

In 1992 Juliette and Adam mounted their own selling exhibition in the house of an architect they had worked with. This was a novel idea in Switzerland but it proved extremely successful. They opened for two days by invitation only to all

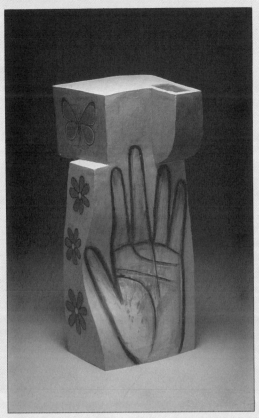

Adam Sutherland,
Ceramic vase,
stoneware, slip
decoration,
tallest 35cm,
1992. Photo:
Stephen Brayne
for the Crafts
Council

their mutual friends and gallery contacts and sold almost all the work exhibited.

They have worked on commissions such as painted tiles and hand-made ceramic sinks. One commission for a stained glass ceiling in a bathroom came from a lady in her 80s who gave them a free hand to determine the budget and design. They have managed to gain private commissions, working in collaboration with architects, during a period when such work was difficult to find in the UK.

Adam and Juliette quote prices in Swiss francs. They find the art business much more professional than in the UK and are rarely asked to provide work on sale or return. The Swiss banking system is efficient and clients transfer payment direct into their account without the need for invoices and reminders. Juliette acknowledges that work commands higher prices in Switzerland. They add a percentage to UK prices for transportation and other expenses.

Juliette Goddard and Adam Sutherland work across many areas in Switzerland: private commissions with architects, exhibiting and selling through galleries and self-promoted exhibitions. They still speak little German or French and conduct all business in English although Juliette recognises that it would be an advantage to learn some German to help in negotiations for commissions.

They got started through a network of family and friends and have concentrated most of their efforts into getting work in Switzerland in the last few years. They began by taking work round the galleries which was a surprisingly positive experience and Juliette says, "I would recommend any young British artist to do it. Swiss gallery owners are very open."

6 • Stay at home – sell abroad

So you have examined your reasons for exporting and are actively exploring ways of networking internationally. At this stage it is worth returning to the question of whether you have put sufficient effort into developing a market for your work at home, firstly for UK buyers and secondly for buyers from overseas.

This second area presents artists and makers with many possibilities for taking what might be described as short cuts to exporting. In other words, making sure the overseas buyer comes to you before seeking them out in their own country. Many artists who have begun to develop an international profile and export their work have started in this way.

The advantages

There are substantial advantages to taking this route. By positioning yourself in a way that brings your work to the attention of overseas buyers or galleries, you will probably be doing a good job in reaching the home market as well. It might be through a trade fair, a high profile gallery or shop, a review or other publicity in a magazine with an international readership or an international slide index. Also, the overseas buyer who comes to you will usually be highly motivated and interested in your work. At a trade fair, for example, where they are in a position to view a huge range of work from this country, it is yours they have selected.

In most cases you are dealing with buyers accustomed to purchasing work in this country. You may find that they will deal with the export formalities or can at least advise you. You can quote your prices in sterling and can usually agree payment in your own currency too. Much of the risk and worry is taken out of the transaction.

A word of warning

However there is one note of caution. If you are considering exporting, it is tempting to make decisions based on which overseas visitors admire and purchase your work in this country.

If, for example, you sell from your studio and notice that French tourists particularly appreciate your work, don't decide that France is definitely the place to export to. Even a direct encouragement such as the American visitor to Chelsea Crafts Fair who confidently pronounces, 'You must sell in Barneys – they love this kind of stuff. You'd do really well there' should be treated with caution. Why? Principally because the French person who finds your studio in mid-Wales or the American who visits Chelsea Crafts Fair is not necessarily typical of his or her compatriots.

The tastes of a well-travelled, cosmopolitan visitor to this country, who may be on a business trip or an independent holiday, are often markedly different from those of local buyers. In fact, you are more likely to attract the interest of these particular buyers by being visible here rather than in their own country. You have the exotic appeal of making something unobtainable in their own country.

So what are the options for presenting your work to the overseas buyer while remaining firmly on your home ground?

Preparation for overseas buyers

Prepare yourself for overseas buyers by thinking carefully about your prices. If you receive an order from an overseas buyer there will be additional costs incurred in getting the work there: shipping, insurance, export documentation and in some cases duty. So you need to be sure you quote the right price and make it clear what is included in it. There are a series of phrases called 'Incoterms' used to describe different ways of quoting prices of work for export depending on what is included. At the least you need to sort out how to quote prices and make sure this appears clearly on any printed wholesale price list you give to buyers.

See page 96, 'How to quote your prices' in 9 • Sales Administration

Don't naively believe that overseas buyers will pay more for the actual work than UK trade buyers. Often they will be more price conscious as there are increased overheads, such as their expenses getting to the UK, to be covered. But do make sure you have included in your prices the increased costs which you inevitably incur in doing business internationally. The cost of phone calls and faxes to confirm

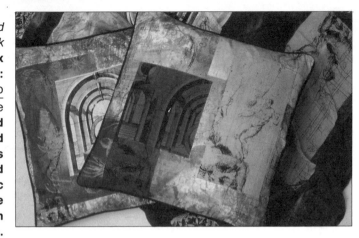

Neil Bottle, *Hand painted silk cushions*, 22" x 22", 1993. Photo: Kate Plumb

Neil Bottle **produces hand printed and dyed silks. His textiles are richly printed with graphic imagery and are used in fashion and interiors. Over several years he has built up a range of export sales, now accounting for 30-40% of his business. He sells to department stores in the United States, Hong Kong, Singapore and Canada and through a gallery in Holland.**

Orders generally come through export buying houses or direct from buyers visiting Chelsea Craft Fair. He is also a member of New Designers in Business which takes a joint stand at various overseas trade fairs. The advantage of this group approach is being able to show work without always having to attend the fair. He has sent work through New Designers in Business to Index 92 in Dubai and IDI Europa in Amsterdam, both major international trade fairs in the interiors and design field.

orders, arrange delivery or chase up payment can mount up. You may have to ring round to get transport quotes or contact courier companies. Additional packaging may be required. There are bank charges for foreign currency cheques.

There may be other things to consider if you are anticipating orders from overseas buyers. For example, is there a label or instructions in English? You might have to produce it in another language. If you make garments which are marked with sizes, they are likely to be different in other countries. Your work might be subject to more rigorous consumer law elsewhere. If an overseas buyer places an order at a UK trade fair, you can expect them to be more familiar with the requirements of their particular market than you are. But check whether they require any modifications to the work or presentation before you agree the order – and the price.

For a fair open to the public you may encounter individual overseas customers. If you are registered for VAT you can offer an added incentive to customers from countries outside the EU with a VAT refund under the Retail Export Scheme.

Trade fairs

There are a large range of trade fairs in the UK and the major ones attract an international clientele. Some are exclusively for trade buyers, others are open to the public.

Trade fairs are mainly of interest to makers although fine artists working in a specialised field such as architecture, those making decorative work for the domestic environment or doing illustration can find them a useful place to present their work. Makers and some fine artists regularly exhibit at fairs such as Top Drawer, the Harrogate Gift Fair, the Birmingham Spring and Autumn Fairs at the NEC and the Ideal Home Exhibition. Chelsea Crafts Fair, where a lot of makers have received their first overseas orders, and the newer Country Living Fair attract a lot of trade buyers and are open to the public too.

Attending a trade fair represents a major investment of time and money although some grants may be available to offset your costs. Try your regional arts board and if you live in a Rural Development Commission area they may be able to help. Buyers visiting trade fairs often expect to see you there a few times before they commit themselves to placing an order. Overseas buyers will need evidence that you are successful and reliable before making that decision.

Research the fair well and ask the organisers for attendance numbers in previous years. If they are interested in promoting the fair as an international event, they can probably give you overseas attendance figures and percentages of export orders taken there.

The right UK gallery

Not many artists feel they are actively targeting overseas purchasers by exhibiting in this country. But some galleries are undoubtedly better at attracting collectors and visitors from other countries and responding to their particular needs. And it isn't just the big name galleries who have an international clientele.

Susie Fisher ran a temporary gallery in a new development of shops in London's Covent Garden. By being in an environment which attracts many foreign visitors, she achieved some success in selling work to them. Susie has developed several interesting overseas opportunities for a number of the artists she represents. These include a commission for a Portuguese client, negotiations with a gallery in Florence for a show of one artist's work and other works commissioned by a German client and for a diplomat in Iceland. When an overseas customer buys work Susie Fisher organises the shipping.

Export buying houses

Export buying houses are agents, generally based in London, who represent the major overseas department stores. Their job is to seek out new merchandise in the UK for their stores to sell. They place orders in this country, organise the shipping and pay you in sterling.

See 12 • Contacts

You can contact export buyers through EXBO, whose members include agents representing leading department stores, such as Macy's and Bloomingdales in the USA and Takashimaya in Japan, Singapore and Sydney as well as importers and manufacturers across the world. Other export buying offices based in London include AGAL, representing Bergdorf Goodman and Neimann Marcus in the USA, Isetan buying for its stores in Japan, Singapore and Hong Kong and the British Isles Buying Agency representing a number of companies.

So dealing with an export buying house is a very easy way of exporting: it avoids the expense and uncertainty of promoting yourself abroad, the agency makes the arrangements for shipping the work, they deal with the export documentation and duties and you don't even have to quote your prices in another currency.

Export buyers are generally oriented towards decorative arts and fashion accessories, eg ceramics, glass, jewellery, textiles, but don't assume that department stores overseas are the same as in the UK. Department stores in Japan often have gallery spaces so the buyers might be interested in fine art and one-off pieces which are suitable for the domestic environment. In 1990 the UK buyer for Macy's in New York decided to set up a Glass Gallery, stocking exclusive one-off pieces, and selected over half the work from UK glass makers.

Rob Turner, who makes exuberantly-decorated bone china tableware, deals regularly with three of the major buying houses, exporting to the USA, Japan and the Far East. He strongly recommends selling through buying houses and says that "once you're tuned into how they work, they are wonderful people to deal with. Buyers have big budgets, are hungry for new work and are always on the lookout for new people." In his experience, the only drawback with export buyers is that you have to be prepared for large orders. It's a 'drawback' many makers dream of but if you aren't geared up to working on that scale, it can be a nightmare. Rob's advice is to be absolutely straight with the buyer about how long it will take to produce the order. It's a good idea to add a margin of time for unexpected delays and, if possible, split the order into several smaller orders.

Textile designer Frannie, who makes hand-painted silk fashion accessories, sells through AGAL. She finds the orders vary from small quantities of work to large orders for mail order catalogues. Many of the top American department stores do mail order and in 1992 she made 3,000 pairs of painted silk cufflinks for Neimann Marcus, ordered through AGAL.

An export buyer may find you if, for example, you exhibit at a UK trade fair or you can approach them direct. This is always worth doing and you need to send good visuals (photographs may be preferable to slides), a price list and concise written information on your work. The next step is usually for them to invite you to the office to show them your work. If you live a long way from London and want to sell through the export houses, it's worth making it clear that you will have no problem bringing your work but, of course, you cannot expect them to cover your travel expenses. When you are a regular on their books, try to persuade the buyers to come to your studio.

As Rob Turner points out, new products are the export buyers' lifeblood. In fact they need you to keep them in work. When you meet the buyers, don't ever say anything negative about your work. Inevitably they always go for the work you like least so just agree enthusiastically that this is one of your favourites too. Buyers are super-professionals when it comes to negotiating deals. But if you are aware that their job is to get your prices down and that your job is to keep them up, the whole process can be quite amicable. A useful response to counter a buyer's call for a lower price is: 'I can't really compromise on the quality, which of course I would have to do to get the prices down.' On the whole, if your prices are fair, US and European buyers won't necessarily expect a discount. So if you do agree a discount, try to trade it for proforma payment. But an experienced designer-maker finds that Middle and Far East buyers always want discounts and recommends you put 5% on your prices to give you the margin to discount.

Rhonda Wilson, *The Magician* (from *Enterprise Heroes* by Rhonda Wilson/Andy Cameron), created from three images: b&w studio portrait of woman, colour picture of desert from visual aids in local library, colour transparency of lilies; scanned onto Syquest disc at 400 dpi and mixed in Adobe Photoshop; output at 800 dpi as 5" x 4" colour transparency; prints made conventionally, 1992.

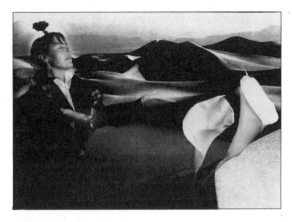

Rhonda Wilson **sees working internationally as an integral part of her work. Her photographic projects are developed as campaigns on social issues such as homeless women and unemployment. This work has come to the attention of overseas gallery curators and she has exhibited in Europe, Australia and the USA. In 1988 'A Sense of Place', an exhibition of images of women and homelessness, was seen in Bradford, London, Rotterdam, New York and Chicago. Interest in the way she works has led to invitations to speak at international photography conferences in Spain and Portugal and at an exhibition of her work in Finland. She is currently working on digitised images which are stored on CD-ROM. New technology offers the scope to send images abroad on disc or via a modem.**

Touring exhibitions

Certain exhibitions in the UK will attract overseas visitors. But the real short cut to exporting is to take part in a touring exhibition which travels to other European countries or further afield.

Sometimes twinning links can be a driving force behind such exhibitions but always make sure that there is a professional level of organisation. It is best if there is a partnership between galleries or museums in the twin towns rather than an arrangement through the town halls. The Usher Gallery in Lincoln toured a mixed exhibition of contemporary craft by 25 Lincolnshire makers to three craft museums in the Rheinland-Pfalz area of Germany, which is twinned with Lincolnshire. A return exhibition toured Lincolnshire. Much of the British work sold and a good quality bilingual catalogue was produced. Two makers received grants to accompany the exhibition and made their own contacts leading to offers of individual shows.

Slide indexes

Some slide indexes have an international remit, whether stated or unstated, while others are designed for regional or local use. If you want your work to be seen by overseas buyers and exhibition curators it is important that you are well-represented with good quality slides of recent work on the right slide indexes.

Jenny Beavan discovered that an American collector used such a route to track down her work. Having read a review of her solo show in the Netherlands, he subsequently came on a trip to London and visited the Crafts Council's slide index to identify which galleries stocked her work. He then travelled down to Cornwall in order to buy a piece from Meridian Gallery near Land's End.

New technology

Of course it's possible to show your work overseas by using electronic technology to transmit the images. It's a neat way of sidestepping all the official exporting channels since you are transmitting documents. In 1990 David Hockney made a large work on paper and faxed it, in A4 sections, to the 1853 Gallery near Bradford. Colour faxes now exist although the quality and permanence of faxed images is often poor.

Rhonda Wilson is also exploring ways of developing her work using computer technology. She creates digitised images which are built up on screen from several images. They can be saved on disk and posted abroad. Digitised images can also be transmitted electronically using a modem. As with fax transmission you need compatible equipment at both ends.

Publicity

There's a range of publicity which can lead to your work coming to the attention of overseas visitors.

If your studio is in a rural or coastal area visited by tourists, concentrate on the tourist information points. The tourist board should have statistics for foreign tourists so try to build up a profile of the overseas visitor to the area. You may decide it is worth producing publicity in other languages to attract such visitors.

Your work or studio might be featured elsewhere, for example on a specialist craft map or general tourist guide. The Wales Tourist Board produce A Touring Guide to Crafts with an introduction in eight different languages, part of their initiative in promoting Wales to overseas visitors.

If you can identify a specialist magazine in your field in another country, you may have some success in placing an article and pictures of your work. You'll need to offer the magazine and its readers something of specific interest. The article could tie in with an exhibition, describe a particular technique you have developed or give insights into the experience of making a living as an artist in your own location. Good visuals can really 'sell' the article to the editor. You could be paid for the article and it may well lead to interest from shops and galleries in that country.

Key points

- There are many opportunities to promote your work in this country which will bring it to the attention to overseas buyers and galleries.
- This way of 'exporting' has many advantages: it is simpler and takes away much of the risk and worry.
- Sales success provides basic export market research and can point the way to which countries to target more directly.
- Beware of making export decisions based on interest from individual overseas purchasers whose taste may not be typical of their compatriots.

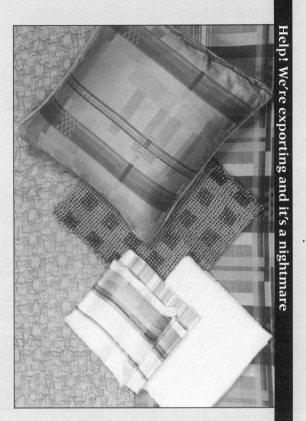

Harriet Wallace-Jones &
Emma Sewell (Wallace
Sewell), **woven textiles,
1993**

**Textile designers and weavers Emma Sewell and Harriet
Wallace-Jones** started trading as Wallace Sewell in 1992.
Soon after this they exhibited their woven fashion and
furnishing accessories at Chelsea Craft Fair. Although they had
not yet begun to develop outlets in Britain, their work attracted
the attention of a number of overseas buyers. They returned
to the workshop with a sheaf of export orders.

The largest orders were from Barneys department
stores in New York and Tokyo. The store sent them a twelve
page instruction manual, the 'Vendor Shipping Package'. For
a first-time exporter it was complex and difficult to understand.
The one thing the manual did make clear was that they would
incur considerable expense if instructions were not followed
to the letter. A few phone calls to New York were necessary to
understand certain points.

So Emma and Harriet tackled a very steep learning
curve when they began exporting. The had to produce five sets

of every invoice and packing list and label each item with the purchase order and style details. To comply with US Customs requirements they sewed fabric labels into each piece with 'Made in England', the fibre content and care symbols.

On one occasion they just missed the shipping deadline. They had understood the 'Latest Shipping Date' noted on the order to mean the date the shipping company collected it from their workshop. However, they discovered it was the date work left the UK (around 4 days after collection).

A particular area of concern was the negotiation of payment terms and discounts. Wallace Sewell quoted prices in Sterling as 'ExFactory', ie without any transportation, insurance or duty included. The shipping company nominated by Barneys collected the cartons from their workshop. But to avoid having to chase unpaid invoices with expensive transatlantic phone calls, they had agreed to payment by letter of credit.

Letter of credit (on sight) guarantees that the money is put aside in the US before the order is dispatched. Once an air waybill has been received as proof of dispatch, it takes around ten days for payment to be transferred into their account. The bank only starts to collect the money on presentation of an air waybill, packing slips, invoices, declaration of country of origin and declaration of correct labelling of goods. A letter of credit costs Wallace Sewell around £120 in bank charges and for such favourable payment terms they had to offer Barneys a discount of 4%. This has been the best solution for large US orders although orders from stores in Japan are on a normal 30 day invoice which is invariably paid on time.

After a year of almost 100% of their business being export, Wallace Sewell realised it was all proving very expensive, worrying and time-consuming. They approached the DTI for assistance and had a free advice session with the area representative. This was very helpful and led to a short consultancy with the Export Development Adviser at the London Chamber of Commerce.

Now they have prepared separate export price lists which take into account the additional administration, packaging and bank charges incurred with export orders. And a more professional approach has freed up time to create new ranges and start promoting their work in the UK. Eighteen months after setting up they are doing around half of their business in Britain, producing ranges for shops such as Browns and Whistles.

7 • Finding your export market

The majority of UK artists and makers currently exporting their work deal with only a small number of countries or trade blocs in the world: notably Europe, Japan & the Far East and North America.

However, even the markets offered within these three blocks are incredibly diverse. You will encounter different ways of doing business, a great diversity of language and culture and a whole series of shifting economic influences. But for these three blocs you are likely to find more information, such as economic reports and guides to business culture, to assist you. And where the path is already trodden by other makers and artists, you can draw on their experience.

Outside these areas artists have of course developed contacts with many other countries, from a trade fair in Dubai to a potter's selling and teaching trip around Australia and an environmental painter's connection with Venezuela. Personal interests and chance encounters are much more likely to foster such links than straight export market research.

The British Council is represented in over 80 countries around the world and can be a good source of advice, contacts and some grants for cultural rather than trade links. The Visual Arts Department in London can put you in touch with the local arts officer in the country you want to work in. Find out whether there are any arts festivals or tours by UK theatre, dance or music companies coming up. If you can time your exhibition with an event like this, you're likely to benefit from the increased publicity and interest in 'British culture'.

When you start exhibiting and selling in other countries, you may find that the overseas gallery's own international networks can further expand your horizons. Links can be based on trading connections, shared language or colonial history. An exhibition in Lisbon, for example, might be the stepping stone to a show in Brazil, while a Madrid gallery could have links with Mexico.

Europe

Europe divides into three areas which require different procedures for export documentation: the European Union countries, the European Free Trade Area and the rest of Europe.

Western Europe is the UK's major trading partner. Being so close, it's easy to find a freight company or you can take work yourself. It is true that for many the English Channel remains a physical and psychological barrier between 'us' and 'Europe'. And since no other stretch of water in the world is as expensive to cross, it can act as an economic barrier as well.

What characterises Europe is its extreme cultural diversity, perhaps as much between the regions as between the countries. Highly sophisticated cosmopolitan cities contrast with underpopulated rural areas. Levels of income and education vary enormously. And there's often a language barrier.

So it would be unwise to decide to 'export to Europe'. Firstly the UK is part of Europe and secondly you'll need to be far more precise and selective about where to concentrate your efforts. There are many readable guides, often found in the reference section of public libraries, which describe doing business in particular European countries and how culture and national characteristics affect it. Most European countries are close enough to plan a 'go and see' trip, taking in some galleries and shops while having a holiday.

There are unexpected differences in the response to UK artists' work. At Trading Places, the seminar on promoting crafts in Europe organised by East Midlands Arts in 1993, Charlotte von Finckenstein shared her experience as director of Galerie L in Hamburg which specialises in glass and ceramics. She finds many British makers use humour in their work which is not well received in Germany. The seminar report sums this up: 'In Germany art is serious. Art is for education. Humour, according to the Germans, does not educate and therefore cannot be sold as an art form.' Charlotte said that collectors in Germany have small flats and therefore have a preference for small pieces. She finds that raku work does not sell well in Germany whereas Nigel Atkins of Galerie du Don in France said that the French liked raku.

Climate, fashion and temperament may lead to other differences in aesthetic preference. For painters, Northern and Southern light will influence how work shows. A jeweller might make large, flamboyant pieces to sell in Spain but be more restrained for Nordic markets.

In marked contrast with the UK, those on higher incomes in most other European countries are interested in owning contemporary art rather than antiques. People aspire to the new rather than the old.

European Union (EU)

Formerly called the European Community, this incorporates the twelve member states: Austria, Belgium, Denmark, Finland, France, Germany, Greece, Republic of Ireland, Italy, Luxembourg, Netherlands, Portugal, Spain, Sweden and the United Kingdom.

Since the establishment of the Single European Market, there is free trade between the EU countries. In fact, there are officially no more exports or imports. Movements of goods are described as 'supplies' and 'acquisitions'.

European Free Trade Area (EFTA)

The seven EFTA countries are Austria, Finland, Iceland, Liechtenstein, Norway, Sweden and Switzerland. These countries (excluding Switzerland) combine with the EU to form a larger trading block called the European Economic Area (EEA).

EFTA countries have a special trade agreement with the EU which means simpler exporting procedures and preferential rates of duty. The DTI publish a clearly-written free guide for exporters covering the EEA, *Trading within Europe,* which contains much useful information.

Eastern Europe and beyond

The remainder of Europe is generally taken to include Eastern European countries, Turkey, Russia, the Baltics and other independent states of the former Soviet Union. Some special trade agreements exist with Turkey.

Since the opening up of the former Eastern bloc, there has been an increased level of contact with artists in Eastern Europe, Russia and the Baltics through exchanges, joint projects and exhibitions. Road freight companies extend far into Eastern Europe, making it easy to find carriers with regular trips to Poland, the Czech Republic, Hungary and beyond.

In terms of selling work, many of these countries accord a high status to artists. The market for art and fine craft has developed rapidly in many former Warsaw Pact countries with the opening up of numerous commercial galleries, often with Western financial backing.

Some countries are developing opportunities for Western artists to exhibit, for example a new international art fair will be held in Prague in 1994. For UK artists and makers, it is possible that direct selling opportunities exist in places with a well-developed tourist trade, such as Prague and other Central European capitals, although it would be hard to get reliable information on local regulations for direct selling. But in general the economies of most Eastern European countries are not yet able to embrace Western prices. Most of the trade in fine art is going in the opposite direction.

North America

This includes Canada and the USA within one trading bloc but in practice most UK artists and makers are exporting to the USA.

America is the world's largest single export market and the second market for the UK. Communications are easy and travel there is relatively cheap. It has a similar-sized population to Europe but with the commercial advantage of a common language and just one currency. The DTI produce a practical guide to doing business in the United States, *Trading with the USA*.

Many artists are enthusiastic about doing business with the States. It's true that economic recession has affected the market in recent years but artists and makers appreciate the refreshingly positive response to their work and a stimulating 'can do' approach to business from the galleries and shops they deal with. US galleries are usually much more geared up to selling than in the UK. Artist Rupert Loydell found that galleries in the States carry a much greater range of work, in terms of both price and quality. He also observed the openness of gallery staff: "You feel you are walking into a selling environment where people want to help you to buy." Attitudes to contemporary art are different too. Sarah Jane Checkland wrote in *The Times* in 1993: "Whereas in Britain less than 10% of wealthy people collect art, in America the figure is 80%."

Specialist galleries and shops are found across the US although there are concentrations in New York, San Francisco, Miami and certain other cities. Buyers for the major department stores and mail order companies visit the Chelsea Craft Fair and major European trade fairs. Many of the stores are represented by export buying houses based in London. Other selling opportunities include good-quality museum shops which sell work by designer makers.

See page 52, 'Export buying houses' in 6 • Stay at home – sell abroad

For the artist or maker wanting to engage with networks in the US, there is a huge range of published opportunities. Magazines such as *American Craft* and the excellent *Art Calendar* ("the business magazine for visual artists") carry substantial listings. You might find requests for work for new galleries and shops, competitions (including a whole section on 'Wildlife stamp competitions' for artists and illustrators), open exhibitions, commissions, residencies, mail art and jobs. American summer schools in the creative arts employ artists and makers to run workshops. Don't expect them to pay your fare when the announcement targets US artists but these jobs are reasonably well-paid and could be the opportunity for an extended selling trip to galleries and shops. Make sure you find out from the US Embassy about whether you need a work permit and always ensure you are fully covered for health insurance.

Japan & the Far East

Japan and certain parts of the Far East (eg Hong Kong and Singapore) offer interesting and lucrative markets. It can sometimes be difficult to find your way in and the language barrier plus the cost of transport almost certainly exclude a 'go and see' approach. Nevertheless, Japanese buyers and collectors do visit the UK. Department stores in Japan are good outlets for fine art as well as craft and many of those in Tokyo, Hong Kong and Singapore are represented by export buying houses in London.

See page 52, 'Export buying houses' in 6 • Stay at home – sell abroad

Because the culture is so different it is worth doing your homework on business and social customs. John Abecasis-Phillips' accessible book *Doing Business with the Japanese* gives plenty of useful background information, describing the Japanese "inherited sense of beauty and refinement, combined with attention to detail, which is all expressed in the products they make as manufacturers and covet as customers". Different customs can lead to new selling opportunities. There is a strong culture of giving gifts: ceramicist Mary Rose Young, who already exports to a department store in Japan, was commissioned to make 70 small vases which a customer ordered as gifts for wedding guests. She finds that orders from Japan are for her most intricate and detailed work: "Customers in Japan want smaller and smaller work while those in the USA want bigger and bigger pieces."

Photographer Susan Derges spent five years in Japan, studying and working. For a while she worked on a Japanese business magazine and notes the very strong emphasis on social bonding in Japanese society between people who do business together. For a foreigner, it is vital to invest a great deal of time on non-business-related activities. Language is an important key to communication and patience and persistence are required in approaching the Japanese market. Susan advised the Photographers' Gallery in

Nick Allen, **glazed entrance doors, wood, pewter, coloured glass acrylic and gold leaf, 3m high, 1993.**

Doors commissioned by a private client in Hong Kong. Over a period of 18 months, Nick Allen **has undertaken four commissions in Hong Kong and made two visits there. He finds the place offers many exciting opportunities but doing business in such a different culture is "a long learning process". Nick has discovered the importance of establishing clear communication channels when dealing with overseas commissions. Because there are several people involved - architect, designer and client, possibly others – he finds it essential to record written details of everything discussed and fax them to all partners. This substantially increases the communications bills and must be costed into the quote. 90% of Nick's work is now overseas. He has private clients in France and had a sell-out exhibition in the United States.**

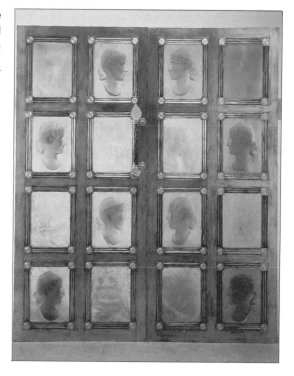

London when they were trying to set up an exhibition and sent letters and faxes to many galleries and artists in Japan without receiving any replies. In fact, Susan reckons that the culture is so different that a direct approach in English is unlikely to work and that personal introductions are often essential to establishing a relationship.

It is worth noting that some parts of the UK have a 'special relationship' with Japan through trading links in the car and electronics industries. In South Wales and Sunderland, for example, you'll find the local authority economic development units have substantial experience of doing business with the Japanese. Language expertise may be available. Where they exist, these local links could be the key to opening up opportunities for exhibitions, exchanges, even commissions in Japan.

Other markets

Infinitely diverse opportunities can be found elsewhere in the world.

Middle East

Some artists have succeeded in the Middle East (eg Dubai and Saudi Arabia) where a special trading relationship with Britain may be of help. There are high-quality trade fairs and you will need to invest in a long-term approach with a market that is extremely wealthy. Culture and religion impose restrictions on women in some countries of the Middle East.

Haggling over price is invariably part of the culture. It happens in shops and trade fairs, even where goods are clearly labelled with the price. Jonathan Andersson, exhibiting at a Dubai trade fair, was advised by the DTI to increase prices by 25%. But he found the customers so expert in hard bargaining that he recommends exhibitors increase prices by 100% to allow for haggling.

Australia & New Zealand

These countries attract many artists and makers. Distance and the size of the markets (the population of Australia is a quarter of Britain's, New Zealand is just over three million) impose limits on trading links. But you'll find a thriving art scene with many galleries and festivals. Cultural diversity and an openness to the new are an intrinsic part of Australian culture and there are many links with the UK.

Potters are particularly interested in Australian ceramics. John Calver enjoyed a rewarding study tour in 1989, meeting many potters on a trip financed through a Northern Arts travel grant, demonstration fees and his own pocket. For his second visit in 1991 he obtained a list of 154 potters groups from the Crafts Council of Australia. A three-month tour, financed by lectures and workshops, was arranged and he met 15 groups around the country, including a week as throwing tutor on the Sydney Ceramic Study Group's annual residential school.

Further abroad

Your interests and contacts may lead you to other countries well off the international art circuit.

Artist Helen Cowcher has made several working trips to Venezuela. Her paintings and successful children's books depicting endangered wildlife species came to the attention of a Venezuelan environmental trust. As a guest of the trust, she stays on their protected ecological estate and spends many weeks painting from nature. Her work has been exhibited in the National Gallery in Caracas.

Photographer Peter Fryer was invited by the British Council in Israel to establish a photography workshop in Nazareth at 'The Arabic Cultural Centre'. Links with Palestinian and Jewish photographers developed into a documentary project on the struggle for Palestinians living in villages within, but not recognised by, the state of Israel. The resulting exhibition toured Israel and North East England. He is now looking to tour the work elsewhere in Europe, the USA, Middle East and Asia.

Key points

- Most artists and makers in the UK who export their work are dealing with just a few countries and trade blocks: notably Europe, Japan and the Far East, and North America.
- Europe is characterised by incredible diversity so you need to be very precise about the country and region you target.
- Many artists find good markets and a good response to their work in the USA where galleries are very geared up to selling.
- In Japan the language and culture are so different you need a high level of patience and persistence to develop contacts. Personal introductions may be helpful and should be cultivated.
- Opportunities elsewhere in the world are just as diverse and interesting. The British Council may be a useful first point of contact for artists seeking to exhibit or develop other cultural links.

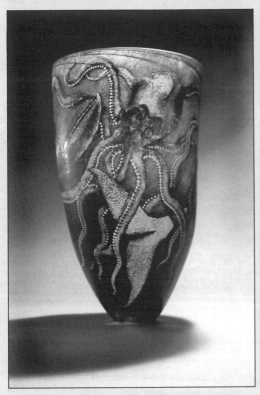

Clare Henshaw,
Sea Dreaming,
**engraved glass
vessel, 42cm x
27cm. Photo:** the
artist

Clare Henshaw is a glass artist, creating finely engraved and coloured one-off pieces. She has exhibited in the Netherlands, Sweden, Switzerland, Germany and the USA.

Clare has established a reputation for her work over a number of years. She finds that because the contemporary glass world is comparatively small, gallery owners tend to approach her for exhibitions. Her work shows in a number of London galleries and is on the Crafts Council's slide index. Living in Bristol, she acknowledges that you need to be visible in certain key places in London to catch the eye of overseas visitors.

Her first major show in the Netherlands was at Rob van den Doel's prestigious gallery in The Hague. It was a successful exhibition, featuring Clare's work alongside that of a Dutch glass artist. Then in 1992 she was invited back to the Netherlands where a solo show at a different gallery in Amsterdam achieved good sales. However, this time she experienced problems and delays in getting the work returned, only getting paid some three months after the exhibition.

But instead of being discouraged she drew up a simple exhibition contract which she now presents to galleries. It sets out the terms and conditions: she agrees to deliver the work and the gallery returns any unsold work. The work must be insured by the gallery once delivered and fully insured on its return journey to the door. Payment must be in sterling and within 30 days of the close of the exhibition. A 10% surcharge is added if payment is made late. The terms of agreement are signed by the artist and the gallery.

Exhibiting in mainland Europe has been an excellent way for Clare to promote her work to collectors. She describes the galleries as "beautiful spaces to show glass" with a much greater choice of specialised galleries than in the UK. They often have much higher budgets for exhibition promotion with good quality full colour posters, private view invitations and cards and prominent advertisements in *Neues Glas*, the influential German glass journal. All these reflect the quality of the work exhibited and help continental collectors take the work more seriously.

Clare Henshaw acknowledges that you do need to persevere in order to establish a reputation in Europe and each show represents a real investment for her. The Art Glass Centre outside Amsterdam where she exhibits in 1994 advise against showing more than once a year in any one European country. Their experience indicates that for a maker of fine one-off art pieces it is preferable to show less frequently and maintain your exclusivity.

She has also begun to promote her work in New York. On a trip to the US she took slides and visited galleries. However nothing concrete came of it. She feels that within the small international glass network, galleries want to have the satisfaction of finding you.

She also made useful professional contacts in the Czech Republic when she wanted to have some large pieces blown. She discovered that this is the only place in Europe with the skill to blow such large pieces. Czech glass artists have developed good working relationships with the glass factories north of Prague. Under the former regime artists were not permitted to have their own workshop equipment and it is still quite common for artists to work within the industry. Clare received a South West Arts award which covered her travel expenses and paid the glassblower's fee for making work to her specifications.

8 • Getting it there

In an ideal world, by the time you take your first export order or accept an invitation to exhibit overseas, you would have researched different ways of transporting your work, identified the paperwork required by Customs, costed up any additional packing material required and worked out insurance values. The real world isn't like that. The chances are you haven't even begun to think about any of it in advance.

But don't panic. There is a series of practical issues to be worked out. The golden rule is to allow yourself plenty of time. It will always take much longer the first time you export. Don't be tempted to cut corners, either in making the work or in making sure it gets there safely.

For a first export order you'll want to impress the customer with your ability to supply work as soon as they require it. Similarly, it would be tempting to accept the earliest date on offer for that long-sought overseas exhibition. But beware of abandoning existing commitments for the sake of pursuing opportunities abroad. And remember that any work you show or sell at a distance must be of the highest possible quality. Overseas customers cannot easily contact you for repairs. Potential purchasers visiting an exhibition will not come to your studio to view a larger range of work. So when you agree a delivery date, allow yourself plenty of time to make the work. That way you can be confident it represents you well.

Export-import

There is a fundamental difference between selling work abroad and selling it in the UK. What you export becomes an import for the receiving country. Documentation is required so that governments can monitor international trade and gather statistics on imports and exports. What for you is a small order for an overseas gallery, is eventually recorded in the balance of payments for two different countries.

While every country is eager to increase its exports, governments may impose certain obligations on goods imported into their countries out of a desire to protect the market for home-produced goods.

Import duty

One of the most important barriers to trade is import duty. This is a tax imposed on goods imported into a country. The rate of duty varies according to the type of goods and is imposed for three main reasons:

- to control imports
- to raise revenue
- to protect local industry.

See page 78, 'International Customs Tariff Code'

Given that these three reasons carry different weight depending on the economic situation of the country, levels of import duty vary around the world. In fact 'works of art' (a category strictly defined by Customs Tariff codes) are exempt from import duty in many countries.

Other barriers to trade

Some of the other ways in which imports can be controlled are by imposing quotas; stringent health, safety and environmental regulations; through subsidies and a whole range of restrictive business practices.

The DTI has a number of Country Desks providing information on import duties and specific regulations affecting imports – ask your DTI Regional Office for the telephone number of the Country Desk required. Alternatively, as the Country Desks are often overloaded with enquiries, you can ring the embassy of the country of destination. Most countries are represented by embassies in London and you should ask for the commercial or information section.

But I'm an artist ...

So what does this have to do with artists? Well, given that the moment you export, your work enters this sphere of import-export regulations, it will come into contact with Customs authorities. They are trained to deal with standard situations and operate according to clear rules. Most of the time they deal with businesses who are familiar with export and import procedures, the sort of businesses with export marketing departments and trained specialists to deal with customs procedures.

Since art is not a standard product, it does not always slot into an obvious category. This can make your life easier or more difficult.

So do take care with any paperwork required and always get advice from the experts. Export advisers, who are based at the main Chambers of Commerce, are very knowledgeable and can usually explain things clearly.

It's worth recording that one artist, who had had some bad experiences of work being held up in Customs abroad, asked a friend who was a Customs officer: "What should I do?" His unofficial advice was: "Art is so difficult. If I were you, I should smuggle it." But of course this book cannot possibly endorse that advice!

Decisions to be made

When you need to get your work abroad, you'll have to research the following areas and make decisions which are right for your particular situation:

- means of transport
- export documentation
- packing the work
- insurance
- any special requirements.

Means of transport

This is also known as shipping. There are many ways of getting your work from A to B. Don't expect to be able to settle on one shipping method to be used in every situation. Different countries and customers will require different solutions.

It's always a good idea to get a range of quotes. You'll need the size and weight of your package as well as the collection and delivery points.

The more information you can provide a transporter with, the more accurate an estimate of costs will be given. Don't forget that for the transporter, the job is a simple physical problem of size and weight. An experienced exhibition organiser reports that the best piece of advice she ever heard was from a cargo handler at an airport: "Remember lady, it's just another piece of freight!" So don't expect any appreciation of the more metaphysical qualities of your work from a shipping company.

Some examples of costs are given below but do remember that the advantages and disadvantages of different methods vary according to the weight and value of the consignment. A light-weight, low-value package can be sent by post while you may find road or sea a better option for a heavy, valuable sculpture.

You will find it convenient to discuss the means of transport at the time you take the order. Sometimes the customer will advise you. Some international competitions specify using a particular carrier. Certain shipping methods allow for cash on delivery so your payment terms may also determine the way you get the work there.

The main means of transport used by artists and makers are the following:

Post

This is usually the cheapest and easiest way of sending work abroad. Ask at the Post Office for leaflets on the Royal Mail International and Parcelforce International services giving charges and weight limits. You can send packages of up to 2kg by letter post and up to 30kg by parcel post. If you have an order which exceeds the weight limit, it may be worth dividing it into several parcels so that you can use the postal service.

Special international services include Recorded and Registered letter post. Recorded is for items of little or no monetary value but Registered post allows you to claim compensation of up to £1,000 and you can also request confirmation of delivery. For Royal Mail services, ask for a certificate of posting. Parcelforce automatically issue receipts.

Parcelforce offer three levels of service for international parcel post which are costed according to speed of delivery. Different levels of compensation apply: the cheapest and slowest Economy service offers limited compensation, Standard service up to £250 per parcel and Datapost up to £5,000 for loss or damage to goods. A special Cash on Delivery service is available for Standard and Economy parcel post.

The Royal Mail leaflet 'Prohibited and Restricted Goods' tells you what goods cannot be sent by post. If in doubt contact your local Customer Service Centre, listed in the phone directory, as different requirements may be imposed by overseas postal services.

Allow plenty of time for work to arrive by post. Apart from the speedy Datapost service, the Post Office can only indicate minimum delivery times. Surface mail parcels can be notoriously slow and some countries are worse than others for delays. Check with the customer whether they recommend you use the postal system. In the USA for example some shops and galleries discourage artists and makers from sending work by post as they do not trust the post, although many artists and galleries do use the US postal system with no problems at all.

Robert Crooks, *Spring jar*,
blown glass, 47cm high, 1992.
In his fourth year of trading as
First Glass, around 60% of
Robert Crooks' **business is
export.** His first American
customers came through the
New York Gift Fair, where he
exhibited in 1992 and 1993.
First Glass now have an
American agent to promote
the work. This arrangement
means that Robert can
package up several orders in
one shipment and send them
via UPS air freight to the
agent's warehouse. The agent
then distributes the work
within the United States. In an
effort to find the right balance
between production and one-
off pieces, Robert has also
exhibited one-off work in fine
art and specialised glass
galleries in the Netherlands
and Germany.

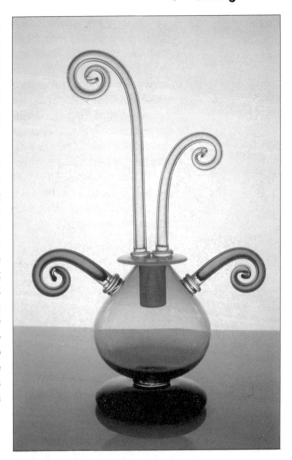

Sample costs using the post

A 2kg parcel costs the following according to destination and
postal or parcel service used:

	Germany	USA
Airmail Small Packet (post)	£3.87	£7.76
Parcelforce Standard Service	£13.70	£17.50

Express delivery services

An extremely reliable way of shipping work overseas is to use an
international express carrier such as UPS, DHL, Federal Express,
TNT, Securicor Omega Express or the Royal Mail's International
Datapost. You can find these through the Yellow Pages under
'Delivery & collection services' or 'Courier services'.

They will usually collect the package from you and give a guaranteed delivery time, for example, next day for Europe and New York, two days for all other countries covered. Of course, you'll pay more compared to sending work by post. But it's hard to beat these services for speed, reliability and convenience. Most importantly, these services reliably track the movement of a package, deal with the customs formalities and guarantee door-to-door delivery. Many makers (of ceramics, glass, textiles, jewellery, etc) find that galleries and shops recommend they use it. The delivery charges are either built into their export prices or billed to the customer.

A firm such as UPS, which is particularly recommended by a number of makers, has the advantage of being internationally known. It can offer a range of services and account facilities which simplify the exporting process.

Sample costs using express delivery services

A 2kg parcel costs the following according to destination and service used:

	Germany (Frankfurt)	New York
DHL	£31.70 (+VAT)	£35.10
UPS	£25.50 (+VAT)	£25.50

Shipping agents & freight forwarders

For larger shipments you may decide to put the work in the hands of a freight company who will take care of transport and customs documentation. You might choose anything from a specialised art transport firm to a general removals company or large international carrier. Air, sea and road are used to get the work there. You can find a shipping company in *Yellow Pages* under 'Shipping & forwarding agents', 'Packers – export' or 'Freight forwarding & storage'. Other general firms with international runs are listed under 'Removals'.

Unlike an international express courier service, your work will probably be consolidated as part of a larger consignment. It is packed and labelled separately but travels as part of a container or lorry load. This means that it is the shipper, rather than you, who determines when work leaves the country. Many firms have regular runs, some specialise in particular destinations. You need to be organised to fit in with their schedule. If you miss their deadline it can mean waiting weeks for space on the next consignment.

Another requirement of shipping companies is for you to advise them of the weight and size (or volume) of the packages some weeks ahead of collection. Carriers do require very accurate dimensions of *packed* works. Three dimensions (height, width and depth) are always required, and at least an approximate weight to enable a company to assess how many people might be required to collect the work. This is necessary to book your space on the consignment but it can be a headache to estimate accurately so far in advance.

Using a shipping firm can be a cost-effective way of sending work overseas. It can be particularly appropriate for large consignments or very heavy work. An experienced firm with a regular run will also be ideal where the work needs to be returned (as with an exhibition).

For exhibitions involving fragile or heavy work it's worth getting quotes from some of the specialist art removers who advertise in *Artists Newsletter* and other fine art magazines. For a cheaper alternative, try a general removals firm. Many have regular runs to mainland Europe. Look for those which specialise in shipping antiques and works of art. They should be expert at moving 'valuables' and 'breakables'. The third possibility is an international freight forwarding company, experienced and widely used for shipping work.

Get a range of quotes and don't be afraid to ask for names of previous customers as referees. You'll need the size and weight of your consignment to get a quote. The quote will generally be by weight and you should also ask about any additional handling charges. Find out whether the company collects from your studio and packs the work themselves. If the work is particularly heavy or your studio is up five flights of stairs, you may be charged extra for collection. Similarly, make sure they know about any access difficulties at the delivery point. If lifting gear is needed to get a large work through an upper storey window because the lift or stairs are too small, this will have a significant impact on the cost of the operation.

When you use an international carrier, check the shipping and delivery times carefully. Always liaise with the shop or gallery receiving the work. If they don't have regular opening times you need to make arrangements for them to be available when work is delivered.

Rail

Few artists and makers consider sending work by rail but the Red Star TCX delivery service is a viable option, covering Western and Eastern Europe, as far as Turkey. Unlike some express delivery services it is available throughout the UK. Goods are collected from your workshop (or you can save £10 by taking them to the station) and delivered to the door in 11 European countries. In 12 others, goods are delivered to selected railway stations. Documentation is straightforward and special insurance cover can be arranged. Jewellery made of precious metals or precious stones cannot be sent by TCX.

> **Sample costs using rail**
> A 2kg parcel costs the following by TCX rail freight according to destination:
>
> | | Germany | Bulgaria |
> | --- | --- | --- |
> | TCX (for up to 5kg package) | £47.00 | £91.00 |

Taking it yourself

In many situations you will want to take the work yourself. It might be for an exhibition, where you want to deliver the work, set it up and attend the private view. You might be taking a vanload of ceramics to sell at a potters' market in Germany or a suitcase of textile samples to show at a US trade fair. There is also the 'gallery crawl' where you plan an itinerary around appointments with galleries and shops.

Taking it yourself is an attractive option, particularly when selling or exhibiting abroad can be combined with seeing something of the country. But keep your priorities straight as holidays and business trips are not always compatible. You'll need to do your homework on what export documentation is required to avoid unexpected delays or expenses when crossing borders. And check out any import limitations: as well as being prepared to pay import duties, there may be restrictions on some goods. In recent years some textile artists have had problems taking silks into the USA.

See page 80, 'Commercial Invoice'

You can carry work with you as part of your baggage when flying, although officially passenger flights are *not* for carrying commercial goods, so airlines are not obliged to help with any customs problems. If goods are being transported under commercial documentation, eg when exhibiting at a trade fair or selling, you need to check them in with Customs on departure and arrival. Report to the MIB (Merchandise in Baggage) office at the airport and allow plenty of extra time.

Certain oil paints and solvents commonly used by artists are banned on airlines. So take care if you are travelling with materials for a painting holiday or to give workshops. Artists have had such materials confiscated by Customs.

You can load up your car and drive there – many do. Probably the only Customs point you'll be stopped at is when you cross the English Channel. Even if you have a van which is clearly identifiable as a commercial vehicle, it's unlikely you'll be stopped until you reach Eastern Europe. But do be aware that if you plan to drive there with a car full of work to sell or exhibit, you are officially considered to be a commercial vehicle. This might mean additional insurance and ferry costs and unless your export documentation is in order, you may spend a long time at customs points.

Be realistic about what you can take on. It may be that the idea of driving down to the South of France is more enticing than the reality. If you're nervous of driving on the right, a long, hot journey carrying valuable, fragile work which your insurance policy states you cannot leave unattended would be no fun. Better to consign the work to a carrier and fly there for the private view.

Artists and makers with experience of taking work themselves recommend travelling with a friend or partner so you can share the driving. Check the ferry routes and choose one which allows you to reach your destination within one day's driving. And if travelling to non-EU countries and carrying goods subject to customs documentation, get expert advice and plan for delays at ports and border crossings.

Documentation

Just as you travel with a passport, so your work will need some form of export documentation. Paperwork required by Customs depends on the country of destination, means of transportation and whether work is being exported permanently or temporarily (as with a non-selling exhibition or samples for a trade fair). "It's a minefield" is the recurring phrase from experts asked for advice on export documentation. But, then again, many artists and makers regularly take and send work abroad with no problems at all. The Single Market has removed Customs formalities within the EU so no special documentation is now required for Member States.

The rules for import/export worldwide are subject to constant change with very little warning. This is especially the case within Europe, and means that it is always worth taking good up-to-date advice from an expert. An individual might find that the more top-of-the-range fine art transport companies are willing to give advice over the telephone.

Sources of advice

Export documentation is a complex area and you should seek advice from a shipping agent or your nearest main chamber of commerce. This is particularly recommended for large consignments and exhibitions since smaller orders are likely to be sent by post or express delivery.

Courier firms provide comprehensive, clear advice and documents for you to complete. Parcelforce has its own straightforward forms but don't count on your local Post Office for reliable information on what paperwork you need to send with packages sent abroad.

Croner's Reference Book for Exporters, which can be consulted in most large public libraries, gives good up-to-date guidance. Unfortunately, the most incomprehensible advice booklets on export procedures can be those produced by HM Customs and Excise. And don't imagine Customs and Excise will tell you how to complete export documents. They state that they cannot tell you what to put down. This covers them in case you make a false declaration. So you'll have to look elsewhere for advice and it may be worth paying an expert to sort it out for you.

The basic requirements

When you are exporting work permanently to countries outside the European Union you need to provide the following documents which are described in more detail in the next section:

Documentation	Who provides it
Commercial invoice	You
Contract of carriage	Freight company
Export documentation (as required)	You or shipping agent
Special declarations or certificates	You (maybe with official endorsement)

When you are exporting work temporarily, and it will *all* return to the UK, the following documentation is required:

Documentation	Who provides it
ATA Carnet	Chamber of Commerce. But you provide the information to the Chamber of Commerce to enable them to draw up the carnet.

International Customs Tariff Code

Also known as the commodity code, this is an internationally-recognised system (the 'Harmonised System') for identifying different types of goods. They are precise multi-digit numbers and are needed for customs documentation when you export to most countries. The code determines the rate of import duty levied.

The best way to find out which codes apply to your work, and if you make a range of different things there may be more than one, is to consult the *HM Customs & Excise Tariff* in a public library. This three-volume reference book lists every type of goods with their corresponding code. It's reasonably easy to find your way around the

SECTION XXI
Works of art, collectors' pieces and antiques

Chapter 97 Works of art, collectors' pieces and antiques

Notes

1. This chapter does not cover:
   (a) unused postage or revenue stamps, postal stationery (stamped paper) or the like, of current or new issue in the country to which they are destined (Chapter 49);

   (b) theatrical scenery, studio back-cloths or the like, of painted canvas (heading No. 59.07) except if they may be classified in heading No. 97.06; or

   (c) pearls, natural or cultured, or precious or semi-precious stones (headings Nos. 71.01 to 71.03).

2. For the purposes of heading No. 97.02, the expression 'original engravings, prints and lithographs' means impressions produced directly, in black and white or in colour, of one or of several plates wholly executed by hand by the artist, irrespective of the process or of the material employed by him, but not including any mechanical or photomechanical process.

3. Heading No. 97.03 does not apply to mass-produced reproductions or works of conventional craftsmanship of a commercial character.

4. (a) Subject to Notes 1 to 3 above, articles of this chapter are to be classified in this chapter and not in any other chapter of the nomenclature.

   (b) Heading No 97.06 does not apply to articles of the preceding headings of this chapter.

5. Frames around paintings, drawings, pastels, collages or similar decorative plaques, engravings, prints or lithographs are to be classified with those articles, provided they are of a kind and of a value normal to those articles. Frames which are not of a kind or of a value normal to the articles referred to in this note are to be classified separately.

1	2A	2B	3	4	5	6	7
97 01 PAINTINGS, DRAWINGS AND PASTELS, EXECUTED ENTIRELY BY HAND, OTHER THAN DRAWINGS OF HEADING NO. 49.06 AND OTHER THAN HAND-PAINTED OR HAND-DECORATED MANUFACTURED ARTICLES; COLLAGES AND SIMILAR DECORATIVE PLAQUES:							
Paintings, drawings and pastels:							
Paintings in oil or water colour	970110 00	1 00		1.Kg 2.Number	Free		S
Other	970110 00	9 00		1.Kg 2.Number	Free		S
Other	970190 00	0 00		Kg	Free		S
97 02 ORIGINAL ENGRAVINGS, PRINTS AND LITHOGRAPHS	970200 00	0 00		Kg	Free		S
97 03 ORIGINAL SCULPTURES AND STATUARY, IN ANY MATERIAL	970300 00	0 00		Kg	Free		S

Example of the International Customs Tariff Codes.
Source: Customs & Excise. Reproduced with the permission of the Controller of Her Majesty's Stationary Office.

index and you must make your own judgement on which category your work falls into.

Works of art come under section 97.01 with various sub-codes depending on materials. In some countries, such as the USA, works of art are not subject to import duty. However, you'd be unwise to dispatch an order of 20 identical ceramic jugs coded as 'original sculptures and statuary'. Customs penalties are high for false declarations.

If you are sending films, videos, photographs or computer disks for exhibition purposes, for a competition or festival, it is not appropriate to classify them as commercial goods. Mark them clearly on the outside: NO COMMERCIAL VALUE – FOR EXHIBITION ONLY, TO BE RETURNED TO SENDER.

Commercial invoice

This is an essential document for exporting. Within the EU it is no longer required but is generally recommended and many express delivery companies insist on it.

The commercial invoice is basically a record of goods and value which you draw up yourself. International delivery firms provide their own forms, which may be called a 'Delivery Note'. But you can easily produce your own commercial invoice, preferably on headed paper. It should be headed 'Commercial Invoice' and list the following details:

- **Sender**: name, address and phone number.
- **Consignee**: name, address and phone number of company receiving the shipment.
- **Full description of goods**: including materials, size, making technique, colour, style description and quantity. For works of art, include the date made and whether signed.
- **Consignment**: number of packages, weight and dimensions of each plus total weight; any shipping marks (ie what is written on packages).
- **Customs Tariff Code(s).**
- **Value of goods:** wholesale value (not the selling price) per item or unit and total value of consignment.
- **Terms of payment.**
- **Sender's and consignee's VAT numbers** (if registered), preceded by appropriate country code.
- **Country of origin**: if destined for an EU country, add "goods in free circulation within the EU".
- **Reason for export.**

wallace#sewell

Emma Sewell Unit 168 51 Clerkenwell Close London EC1R 0AT
Telephone/fax 071 251 1143 VAT No. 627 401 361

INVOICE

TO: Lady Penelopes
Parker Court
686 Fifth Avenue
New York, N.Y. 10023

FROM: Emma Sewell

TAX POINT: 31 March 1994
INVOICE NO: 94/28
PURCHASE ORDER NO: 305466
VAT NO: 627401361

DEPT: 2305   **TERMS:** EX-FACTORY - LC SIGHT

38 WOVEN SCARVES

VENDOR STYLE	STYLE DESCRIPTION	COLOUR DESC.	FIBRE CONTENT	UNIT PRICE	QUANT.	TOTAL
ES/LSEW	EXAGG WEAVE	BROWN/GOLD	50% SILK/50% LINEN	£48.00	3	£144.00
ES/LSEW	EXAGG WEAVE	IVORY/STONE	50% SILK/50% LINEN	£48.00	3	£144.00
ES/LSEW	EXAGG WEAVE	POWDER BLUE/GREY	50% SILK/50% LINEN	£48.00	4	£192.00
ES/LSEW	EXAGG WEAVE	VICT PINK/GRY GRN	50% SILK/50% LINEN	£48.00	4	£192.00
ES/LSDC	DOUBLE CLOTH	BROWN/GOLD	75% SILK/25% LINEN	£48.00	3	£144.00
ES/LSDC	DOUBLE CLOTH	IVORY/STONE	75% SILK/25% LINEN	£48.00	3	£144.00
ES/LSDC	DOUBLE CLOTH	BARLEY/MUSHROOM	75% SILK/25% LINEN	£48.00	4	£192.00
ES/LSDC	DOUBLE CLOTH	POWDER BLUE/GREY	75% SILK/25% LINEN	£48.00	4	£192.00
ES/LSGP	GAP STRIPE	CAYENNE/PEWTER	75% SILK/25% LINEN	£48.00	3	£144.00
ES/LSGP	GAP STRIPE	IVORY/STONE	75% SILK/25% LINEN	£48.00	3	£144.00
ES/LSGP	GAP STRIPE	VICT PINK/GRY GRN	75% SILK/25% LINEN	£48.00	4	£192.00

SUB-TOTAL: 38   £1824.00

DISCOUNT FOR LC: 4%   £ 72.96

TOTAL: £1751.04

LATEST SHIPPING DATE: 30 APRIL 1994
PAYMENT TERMS: LC SIGHT
BANK: Barclays Bank PLC, Barclays Business Centre, 193 Clerkenwell Road, London EC1, U.K.
ACCOUNT NAME: Wallace Sewell   **ACCOUNT NO:** 20945842   **SORT CODE:** 20-17-68
COUNTRY OF ORIGIN: England

Any charges/expenses/deductions incurred by the vendors - WALLACE SEWELL - due to errors made
by the Purchasers, their bank or parties in their employ will be borne by the Purchasers.

SIGNED:

Sample invoice used by Wallace Sewell to send work to the USA

You need three copies of the commercial invoice and each should be signed (with an original signature) and dated. For certain types of payment, eg letter of credit, you will need a fourth copy. It's certainly worth having spares – just in case!

Don't forget that the commercial invoice is not necessarily the same as your invoice for payment, although it contains much of the same information. The commercial invoice is used where goods may be sold or not. For example, you would draw up a commercial invoice when sending samples to a trade fair. In that case the consignee would be the fair organisers, although they are obviously not purchasing the goods. The commercial invoice would state 'Trade Samples for exhibition and sale at the ABC Trade Fair, or return to the United Kingdom' as the reason for export.

Outside the EU and EFTA countries import duty and taxes may be levied. Since these are worked out as a percentage of the quoted value, it is in your interest to keep the value as low as is

wallace#sewell

Emma Sewell Unit 168 31 Clerkenwell Close London EC1R 0AT
Telephone/fax 071 251 1143 VAT No. 617 401 961

PACKING LIST

TO: Lady Penelopes
Parker Court
686 Fifth Avenue
New York, N.Y. 10023

FROM: Emma Sewell

TAX POINT: 31 March 1994
INVOICE NO: 94/28
PURCHASE ORDER NO: 305466
VAT NO: 627401361

DEPT: 2305   **TERMS:** EX-FACTORY - LC SIGHT

38 WOVEN SCARVES

VENDOR STYLE	STYLE DESCRIPTION	COLOUR DESC.	FIBRE CONTENT	UNIT PRICE	QUANT.	TOTAL
ES/LSEW	EXAGG WEAVE	BROWN/GOLD	50% SILK/50% LINEN	£48.00	3	£144.00
ES/LSEW	EXAGG WEAVE	IVORY/STONE	50% SILK/50% LINEN	£48.00	3	£144.00
ES/LSEW	EXAGG WEAVE	POWDER BLUE/GREY	50% SILK/50% LINEN	£48.00	4	£192.00
ES/LSEW	EXAGG WEAVE	VICT PINK/GRY GRN	50% SILK/50% LINEN	£48.00	4	£192.00
ES/LSDC	DOUBLE CLOTH	BROWN/GOLD	75% SILK/25% LINEN	£48.00	3	£144.00
ES/LSDC	DOUBLE CLOTH	IVORY/STONE	75% SILK/25% LINEN	£48.00	3	£144.00
ES/LSDC	DOUBLE CLOTH	BARLEY/MUSHROOM	75% SILK/25% LINEN	£48.00	4	£192.00
ES/LSDC	DOUBLE CLOTH	POWDER BLUE/GREY	75% SILK/25% LINEN	£48.00	4	£192.00
ES/LSGP	GAP STRIPE	CAYENNE/PEWTER	75% SILK/25% LINEN	£48.00	3	£144.00
ES/LSGP	GAP STRIPE	IVORY/STONE	75% SILK/25% LINEN	£48.00	3	£144.00
ES/LSGP	GAP STRIPE	VICT PINK/GRY GRN	75% SILK/25% LINEN	£48.00	4	£192.00

SUB-TOTAL: 38   £1824.00

DISCOUNT FOR LC: 4%   £72.96

TOTAL: £1751.04

COUNTRY OF ORIGIN: England
NET WEIGHT: 3.5 KG
GROSS WEIGHT: 3.9 KG

Sample packing list used by Wallace Sewell **to send work to the USA**

reasonable. It is not uncommon for makers, overseas galleries, shops and advisory bodies to suggest you undervalue your shipment in order to reduce duty. However you should be aware that goods are only insured in transit for the value quoted and that false customs declarations incur severe penalties. Similarly, where duty is not payable, you would be unwise to overinflate values.

As well as sending a commercial invoice when others are transporting your work, you can use it when you carry goods through Customs yourself. Jane Adam uses a commercial invoice when taking her jewellery samples into the US for trade fairs. When leaving the UK she takes the three copies to the Customs desk at Heathrow Airport. Officials check the paperwork and goods, keep one copy and stamp another to confirm it has been inspected. At New York Customs, Jane passes through the Red Channel. US Customs officials check goods in on the computer, calculate duty (around 10% for jewellery) and take payment, which can be by credit card.

However, on a recent trip, Jane discovered there is a limit (currently around $1700) on the value of goods which can be imported by an individual as 'merchandise in baggage' (MIB). If your goods are over this limit, you need to ship goods into the country by some other method, eg post, air freight or shipping company. On this occasion, the value of her samples took her over the limit, so Customs issued a Carnet allowing temporary admission of the goods which detailed every piece. Jane would normally sell her samples at a trade fair but this is not permitted with a Carnet and everything was checked on departure from the US. Jane Adam recognises that Customs were under no obligation to issue a Carnet so that she could clear the samples into the country. It was only because her paperwork gave tariff numbers and values, and therefore made it easy for them, that they agreed to do so.

If carrying valuable work yourself to countries outside the EU, it is advisable to check whether there is a limit for such imports (known as 'merchandise in baggage'). Try asking the DTI country desk or the commercial section of the relevant embassy. It is not normally possible to obtain a Carnet on arrival and if you are over the limit you might find yourself facing an expensive bill to get a customs agent to sort the problem out for you.

Contract of carriage = proof of export

The document given to you by the freight company which acts as proof of dispatch is officially known as the contract of carriage. This document carries much the same information as the commercial invoice. It has different names according to the means of transport: Bill of Lading for transport by ship, Consignment Note or CMR for road freight, CIM for rail freight and an Air Waybill for goods sent by air. If you send work by post, ask for a certificate of posting (issued free) which acts as the proof of export.

When goods are transported by ship, the bill of lading also acts as a title document conferring ownership, and must be transferred to the person receiving goods so that they can claim them at the other end.

The main reason for keeping your copy of the contract of carriage is if goods are subsequently returned to the UK. Then you have to produce the document in order to recover them. The document acts as 'proof of export' to satisfy Customs that the goods are not being imported. In this situation, goods are technically called 're-imports'. If a shop or gallery returns work to you from overseas which has previously been exported, instruct them to mark the package clearly 'British Returned Goods'. This avoids your having to pay duty or tax on the package when it clears UK Customs.

Richard Allen, **charcoal on paper, 1993**

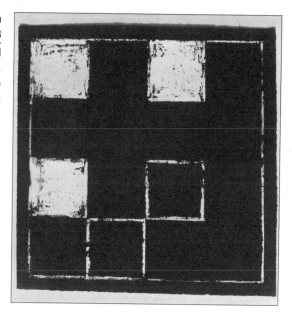

Richard Allen has exhibited work abroad for many years. One man shows include Gallery del Cavallino in Venice, Rijkscentrum Hoger in Brussels, the Basel International Art Fair in Switzerland, Gallery Takagi in Japan and Printworks Gallery in Chicago. His work is represented in many overseas public collections including National Academy of Art, New Delhi; Museum of Modern Art, Rome; Museum of Modern Art, Rio de Janeiro; the Lodz Museum, Poland and the University of Vermont, USA. In the 1970s, before the establishment of the Single European Market, getting stuck at Customs en route for Belgium and Holland was a frustrating and sometimes expensive part of the process. He has shown in the USA in recent years and regularly sends prints to a gallery in Chicago. Richard finds the simplest way of getting work there is to send it by post in a tube. He sends prints, drawings and gouaches this way and arranges for the gallery to frame work in the States.

Special export documentation

This is where it can start to get more complicated. If a shipper is transporting work for you, they will probably be the agent who draws up documentation for the total consignment. If, however, you are taking work yourself and travelling outside the European Union, get up-to-date guidance from the export section of your local Chamber of Commerce.

The purpose of the documents is two-fold. They act as a record for overseas trade statistics and are also used to obtain preferential rates of duty in some countries.

The two most common documents used are the Single Administrative Document (appropriately called the SAD form) and the EUR1 Movement Certificate. Both are available free from Customs. You should ask to speak to the 'paperkeeper' and always ask them to supply the explanatory leaflets as well as the customs forms.

The Single Administrative Document is used for customs entry and statistical purposes for trade to all parts of the world. The full SAD procedure is not always necessary for exports. It is required if you are transporting work yourself which will be sold *except* in any of the following circumstances:

- when goods are covered by an ATA Carnet
- when goods are below a certain value
- when goods travel under a contract of carriage, eg air waybill.

Export advisers proudly announce that the SAD document replaces some 70 export documents that existed previously. Nevertheless it is a pretty daunting form and the explanatory notes are not easy to understand. But if you have already made out a commercial invoice, you have all the information you need to complete the SAD form. It's worth getting it checked by an expert at the Chamber of Commerce.

The Movement Certificate EUR1 is used for sending work to EFTA countries and some others (eg Cyprus, Malta, Israel). It proves that the goods originate from a European Union country. This ensures that no duty is payable within EFTA countries and preferential rates are applied in other countries covered by the EUR1 form.

For some countries, particularly the Middle East and South America, the Chamber of Commerce warns that a lot of export documentation is required. Documents must be legalised by the embassy before goods are shipped and it can be very expensive.

Declaration or Certificate of Country of Origin

Goods exported outside the EU generally require this declaration. You can draw it up yourself on headed paper, giving all the references which identify the goods, ie the invoice number and consignee plus purchase order number and any other goods reference numbers. You then make a statement, eg:

'For shipments covered by Invoice: 118
We declare that the country of origin referred to in the invoices quoted above is the UNITED KINGDOM.'

Sign and date the declaration and send three copies. Keep the original.

The declaration should be accurate and reflect the country of origin of the materials as well as the making. However, you can complicate your life by getting too detailed about every component. In some places, mention of certain countries of origin is liable to lead to goods being delayed by Customs. The US is particularly sensitive about silk imports from the Far East, and don't send goods originating from or made of materials from Taiwan to Korea.

This document is also commonly known as the Certificate of Country of Origin. Most countries you are likely to deal with accept the use of a standard form CVO (Combined Certificate of Value and

Origin) – see *Croners Reference Book for Exporters* under the relevant country. If some other type of Certificate of Origin is needed, it can be arranged through your local Chamber of Commerce for a fee.

Other declarations & certificates

Find out from the DTI country desk or embassy whether any other declarations or certificates are required. For the USA, for example, ceramic tableware requires a statement that it "complies with the acceptable standard to lead and cadmium release laid down by the US FDA".

Wallace Sewell were advised they had to make a declaration that "the merchandise is legally marked to conform to US trade commission and US customs regulations".

ATA Carnets

ATA Carnets are issued for goods to be exported on a temporary basis, eg for an exhibition or for samples for a trade fair, where the goods will be re-imported. The Carnet acts as a bond which enables goods to pass through customs without payment of duty or tax. The Carnet is *not* suitable where some work may sell or remain overseas. The categories of goods which may travel under a Carnet are defined by International Convention and include 'Commercial Samples; Goods for International Exhibition; Professional Equipment: Articles; ... to promote any branch of learning; art; craft ....' Carnets are issued by Chambers of Commerce who charge a standard fee of £110, reduced to a minimum of £65 for Chamber members.

To issue a Carnet, the Chamber needs a detailed list of everything going out, with valuations and country of origin. They need to know all the countries to be visited, including those the goods will pass through and the dates of departure and return. A Carnet is valid for a maximum of one year and can cover a touring exhibition visiting more than one country as long as the entire route is pre-determined.

It's best to keep the values low since you have to give the Chamber of Commerce a deposit which is equivalent to the duty and tax payable if the goods were exported. This deposit acts as a bond or 'counter indemnity'. It's usually in the form of a bank guarantee but sometimes you have to pay over a cash deposit – the Chamber can advise you which is best for your situation.

But again, be realistic in placing a value on the goods since you cannot insure the consignment for more than the stated value. When the goods come back to the UK and you return the fully endorsed Carnet to the Chamber of Commerce, this deposit is returned. If the total shipment does not come back, you can forfeit all or part of the financial bond. In this situation, the Chamber will be presented with a bill for duty and taxes by the overseas government; they can only pass on that bill to you and use all or part of the deposit to pay it.

Jenny Beavan sent some work to Istanbul under a Carnet for an exhibition. She had to open a special building society account with £800 in it as a deposit (the total value of the shipment was around £2,000). She was required to keep the deposit in this account for some time after the goods had returned 'in case Customs want to make a claim'.

Export licences

The reason why goods described as 'Works of Art' may attract Customs attention is because certain works of art require an Export Licence to leave the country. UK and EC licences are issued by the Department of National Heritage who can provide a leaflet, *Guidance to Exporters of Cultural Goods* stating where they are required.

Export Licences are only needed for works over 50 years old which exceed a certain value, eg original sculptures more than 50 years old and valued at over £39,600. The minimum value for works requiring an Export Licence is £6,000 (for photographs, textiles and portraits of 'British Historical Persons', again only works created over 50 years ago). So even if you use old objects in your installation work, you are very unlikely to come under the Export Licence requirements.

Post Office customs declaration

The Post Office supply small green Customs declaration forms for packages going outside the European Union. If goods are marked as gifts or samples (ie they have no commercial value) they are not exports and incur no duty. However commercial goods sent by post should also carry the appropriate export documentation, ie a commercial invoice and any certificates required. You should state the weight and value on the green Customs form.

For some countries of destination, eg the USA, Customs authorities only collect import duties on postal packages over a certain value. It's worth finding out about this from the commercial section of the relevant embassy as it can make sending small consignments of goods by post a cost-effective option, for you and the overseas customer.

Packing slips

These may be required if sending work to an overseas department store or chain of shops. There are needed to help the store identify and distribute the goods and to help Customs and the freight company identify what goods are in each package. Packing slips must be drawn up accurately, and list the goods contained in each carton with all reference numbers. You usually need to send several copies and keep the original in case of query. Copies of the packing slips are required to clear payment by letter of credit.

Packing the work

However you decide to ship the work, it is vital to pack it extremely carefully. If your prices state 'plus packing', you can charge the customer a reasonable amount for any special cartons, labels or padding materials you have to purchase.

Assume the worst. A package covered with fluorescent 'Fragile' and 'This Way Up' labels may be dropped or travel upside down with a heavy weight on top of it. Extremes of temperature and humidity will affect some work so make sure the packaging is substantial enough to protect it from the elements. Address labels should be written with a permanent marker pen and affixed with both glue and sellotape. Many mail order companies put the delivery documents in strong plastic envelopes stuck on the outside of the parcel.

In addition to possible damage in transit, the package may be opened for examination by customs authorities. It's worth anticipating this in the way you pack the work. You may want to mark it with instructions for opening and re-sealing. This can be as simple as FRAGILE, OPEN THIS END, THIS WAY UP.

For exhibition work, it will usually be cheaper and safer to send work unframed and get the gallery to organise framing when it arrives.

If you are using a freight forwarder or removals firm, they often supply their own crates and pack work themselves. You should always supervise the process. In the case of damage in transit, you will be better protected under their insurance policy if they have packed the work. Their packing crates are a standard size to simplify loading and unloading.

Insurance

It is wise to check the insurance cover for goods in transit. Cover provided by your own household or studio policy is likely to be minimal unless you take out a special policy. Glassmakers Catherine Hough and Steven Newell, trading as Victoria Glass, supply shops and galleries in Europe, Japan and the USA. They have their own insurance policy which covers loss or damage anywhere in the world. However, many artists and makers take out insurance for individual shipments which is quite straightforward. There are a number of areas to consider.

Goods in transit

Goods should be fully insured for loss or damage for the whole of the journey. Cover may also be offered for 'consequential loss', eg where you lose orders in the event of work not arriving for a trade fair.

Shipping companies can quote insurance rates for a consignment. Courier firms and postal services detail standard maximum rates of compensation and you can pay a supplement for extra cover. If the goods are particularly valuable it may be better to split the shipment into several packages.

The most difficult situation to get full cover for is when you are taking work yourself. Holiday travel insurance policies may exclude business trips and motor insurers are very cautious about cover for goods left unattended in a vehicle.

In 1992 the Quay Arts Centre on the Isle of Wight organised an ambitious exchange exhibition with partners in Spain, Portugal, Germany and Denmark. They sent a vanload of work by Isle of Wight artists around their partner galleries in Europe to deliver work and collect pieces for a European exhibition at the Quay Arts Centre. Space on the van was limited as the two organisers had to sleep in it because insurance cover for unattended goods was not available!

In all cases, check the maximum compensation per article and make sure it is high enough. Don't forget that you can only claim for any losses against the stated value on your commercial invoice or ATA Carnet.

Green Card

If driving in Europe with your work, you'll need a Green Card to extend your vehicle insurance cover. Ring your motor insurance company in advance and give them the dates of your trip and countries to be visited. Insurers don't usually charge for these but if you have a commercial policy there is likely to be a charge.

Potter Chris Speyer, trading as Yerja, travelled to the Diessen ceramics market in Southern Germany. As the company has a commercial insurance policy on their van, they were charged around £90 for a week's Green Card.

Sub-contracted delivery firms

Large shipping companies are usually based at ports and airports. They often sub-contract the collection of your goods to a local delivery firm. In this case it's worth checking your work is properly insured while in their care.

Textile artist Neil Bottle was concerned when a valuable consignment of work, bound for America, was collected by a local pick-up company in a dodgy-looking van. To his horror he discovered that insurance cover for that part of the journey would only be on a weight basis. His hand-painted silk accessories would be covered for only a fraction of their true value. The local carrier even planned to leave the goods in his van overnight before taking it to Gatwick. Neil immediately arranged to pay an insurance supplement to give him proper cover.

Liability insurance for exporters

Few makers or artists even consider this. However, a textile artist who exports regularly to the USA recently changed his insurance company. When the broker went over all the areas of business requiring cover, the artist was informed that his new insurance policy included a special supplement for £300 per year. This covers him for potential legal or public liability claims resulting from doing business with the USA. However, jeweller Jane Adam's insurance broker told her not to bother with liability insurance for exports. Insurance brokers' advice clearly varies. It should be based on your product, your volume of business and the statistical likelihood of any claims.

Personal insurance

When you are travelling abroad always make sure you have adequate insurance cover for healthcare and your personal baggage. If you are travelling within the European Union, you should take form E111 (available from any Post Office). This covers you for general and emergency care although in some countries you need to pay for treatment and claim a refund when you return to the UK.

A holiday insurance policy may seem the obvious choice for full cover but do read the small print carefully to make sure there are no exclusions for business travel. It's worth investigating the cost of proper business insurance cover which should ideally include cover for consequential loss, such as loss of business if you were unable to attend a trade fair. Ask your insurance company or an insurance broker.

Exhibitions and competitions

This is another area notoriously difficult to get adequate insurance cover for. When sending work overseas for an exhibition, do check that it will be covered under the gallery's policy – for loss or damage on display, when setting up and in storage.

If you are organising your own exhibition in a non-gallery venue, insurance may be impossible to arrange. In this situation, pay special attention to security and invigilation.

Competitions and open exhibitions set their own conditions for insurance of works submitted. These often advise you that the organisers will accept no liability and you should arrange your own insurance. Try your own insurers or a broker but you may find it is impossible to get cover for a situation outside the UK where you can give no guarantees on levels of security or care. If in doubt, ask the organisers to give you names of UK artists who participated in previous years and who may be able to reassure you on the professionalism of the event and the organisers.

Ceramics artist Jenny Beavan found that the renowned International Biennial at Vallauris states that work is insured during the exhibition but not for the period it is stored after delivery by the carriers. She went as far as Lloyds of London in her quest for insurance cover but none was available. So she had to trust to the professional competence of the organisers of the event.

Special requirements

When exporting you should always check whether the country of destination requires any special labels or modifications to your work. This is so that it conforms to both Customs and local consumer legislation. Ask the customer, the DTI and any specialist trade association you belong to for guidance. Do not neglect these requirements as a missing label or instruction booklet may make the goods illegal and unsaleable.

Health and safety legislation on consumer goods is likely to be different elsewhere. It is particularly stringent in the USA. Get specialist advice if you produce work for the domestic environment where special labelling of flammable fabrics, lead content in glass, composition of ceramic glazes etc may be required.

Many countries require goods to have a 'Made in England' label or sticker and you may have to order these in advance and attach to every item. If your work normally carries instructions, find out whether you are obliged to produce these in the language of the destination country.

Another example of a special requirement would be the labelling of textile goods which should carry appropriate care instructions using the international symbols. Toys and electrical goods are also subject to special labelling and licences according to the country of destination. Hallmarking requirements and descriptions of metals may be different elsewhere.

You should also consider whether your imagery is likely to face censorship in the country of destination. Work which deals with sensitive issues such as politics, religion or sexuality may be banned or even destroyed.

Dealing with problems

In the event of any delays or difficulties you will need the export documents (commercial invoice, packing slips, air waybill, etc) so keep them in order.

The most common problem is for goods to be held up at Customs and this can happen for a variety of reasons. This is why you should always allow plenty of time. Jonathan Andersson has exhibited at a number of overseas trade fairs. When travelling to the Miami Art Fair, the shipper advised him that his work would take seven days to arrive. He therefore covered himself by sending it out there seventeen days ahead of the event. He also planned to arrive three days in advance to give him time to deal with any problems which might arise.

If work is held up or lost in transit, respond quickly and decisively and press the shippers or airline to find it as a matter of urgency. Textile designer Gordana Mandic travelled to the San Francisco Gift Fair but her work was lost en route. As she was travelling as part of the British Exhibitors' delegation with the Crafts Council, she immediately informed the British Consulate who she found very helpful. They contacted the airline on a number of occasions until the case was located and flown to San Francisco. She then encountered problems with Customs clearance and because of the need to clear the work quickly for the Gift Fair, she had to engage an official customs broker. There was a substantial bill for this agent's services and she is negotiating with the airline for compensation.

If you do encounter problems with Customs clearance, the advice from Sue Webber, export adviser at the Bristol Chamber of Commerce is "grovel"! She always encourages companies to take a humble attitude with customs authorities and ask for their advice on how the problem can be sorted out. The power of the individual customs officer should never be underestimated. It is easy to hire one of the experienced Customs agents who are based at airports and ports, to speed up clearance of your work. Ask at Customs for a list of registered agents. Find out what the charges are likely to be before you commit yourself. Certain commercial insurance policies would offer cover for loss of business arising from such delays.

Key points

- International trade is regulated by procedures laid down by countries in order to monitor their imports and exports. Customs codes are used to identify types of goods and import duties may be levied.

- Goods can be sent by post, air freight, road carrier, ship or rail. Carrying goods with you is often the best solution but it may be subject to certain restrictions and the paperwork may be more complicated.

- The documentation required for Customs clearance must be prepared accurately and with multiple copies.

- Insurance is an important consideration when deciding how to send work. It is vital to ensure that work is fully covered in transit in the event of loss or damage.

- Robust packaging and clear labelling is essential for the safe passage of your goods from one country to another.

- The rules for import/export worldwide are subject to constant change with very little warning, so always take good up-to-date advice from an expert.

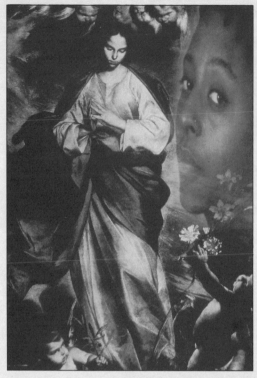

Roshini Kempadoo, *A Bit of the Other – No. 8,* **dyesublimate print from computer-generated image, 1993.**

Roshini Kempadoo is a free-lance photographer who has developed an international reputation through her work over the past few years.

In 1991 she spent some time in the USA on internships working at the National Museum of African Art in Washington and the Schomberg Center for Research into Black Culture in New York. Her connection with the USA continued with work selected for group shows including *Disputed Identities* at San Francisco Camerawork and *Interrogating Identities,* a touring exhibition curated by Kelly Jones for the Grey Art Center in New York. She has given guest lectures in Washington and New York.

In 1990 her work was featured in *Art Forum* journal. A Dutch curator noted the review with interest and as a result Roshini was offered a one woman show at Gallery Perspektief in Rotterdam. The show, *Roshini Kempadoo – Culture and Identity,* was successful and included a guest lecture at the gallery. A portfolio of Roshini's work was published in *Perspektief,* a Dutch photography magazine, as part of the exhibition agreement.

Since then she has been commissioned to produce a body of work for the Oude Kerk Stichting, an art foundation based in a church which has a high profile exhibition programme in Amsterdam. The brief was to document and produce a series of images on the areas and communities surrounding the church, situated in the middle of the red light district. The fee covered a week's work plus expenses. It was a particularly challenging commission as Roshini found it almost impossible to photograph anything – the prostitutes, pimps and clients who throng the district did not wish to be identified. The final work, *A Bit of the Other,* is a series of photo-compositions made up of reportage-style photographs and computer-generated images which take the viewer on an uncomfortable journey around notions of desire and power. The work culminates in a photographic publication and exhibition in Amsterdam in 1994.

Roshini Kempadoo views developing her international work as a long-term process which is necessary to establishing oneself as a practitioner. Slowly but surely the work comes in. Galleries, museums and the occasional private collector buy work and with new commissions she always tries to negotiate the purchase of a piece prior to accepting the commission. But she accepts that international work often represents a substantial personal investment. Exhibition fees for artists are not the norm in the USA or the Netherlands. Phone calls and faxes to the USA to negotiate materials and transport costs are at her own expense. Where possible, she tries to send work unframed.

She has found that her work has been seen by overseas exhibition curators through UK slide indexes and picture libraries with an international sphere of influence. She advises photographers to be aware of this when deciding where to place their slides since some indexes are of national or regional interest only. Her slides are with AXIS, Autograph, the Women's Artists Slide Library and, as a Format photographer, she is well represented in the Format Partners Photo Library. She has also found that international networking between curators often tends to bypass the UK. Despite having successful exhibitions in Britain, it was only when she was featured in *Art Forum* and other international magazines and publications that she came to the attention of a Netherlands gallery.

9 • Sales administration

Selling your work abroad involves additional time and expense so your prices need to allow for this. As well as the obvious costs incurred in shipping work overseas, there may be hidden expenses – bank charges for clearing foreign payments, special labels, translation fees, expensive phone calls and faxes to confirm orders and chase payment as well as losses if currency exchange rates go against you.

Plan for such expenses through the way you quote prices and accept payment. There are many different options for each. Ideally you'll need a clear understanding of these before you start taking export orders. All too often the customer dictates the payment terms so you probably can't apply one system to all export situations. But it will make your sales administration simpler if you try and establish some consistency in the way you deal with overseas sales.

How to quote your prices

The first thing to sort out is how you quote your prices. There are a series of standard expressions called 'Incoterms' which are shorthand ways of describing what is and isn't included in the price quoted.

ExWorks. Many makers quote their prices ExWorks (or ExFactory). This means the basic price as if the goods were collected from your studio. ExWorks prices exclude transport, insurance in transit and duty where payable.

FOB: free on board. If you live within range of a major port or airport, you might want to quote prices FOB. This means that you bear the cost and responsibility for transporting work to the point of departure. For a port, eg 'FOB Southampton', you would pay any charges necessary to load the consignment onto the ship. For an airport, eg 'FOB Gatwick', you merely need to deliver goods to the air freight company.

C & F: cost and freight. You pay for the shipping charges and any other expenses necessary to get the work to an agreed destination, eg 'C & F San Francisco'.

CIF: cost, insurance and freight. As with C & F plus you cover the insurance costs for goods in transit.

Delivered Duty Paid. You organise delivery of the goods to the customer and cover all costs for transport, export administration, insurance and any duty and taxes payable. This makes the order as easy for the customer as ordering from a local supplier.

Which one to choose

So why choose one rather than another? In some cases the buyer will dictate the terms, often where they do all their business in the same way. ExWorks is certainly the easiest and is preferred by most makers. However, in order to reach certain buyers it is worth considering other ways of quoting your prices. Jane Adam sells to many small galleries and shop in the USA and has found that Delivery Duty Paid is the only way to attract such business. The buyers are not accustomed to dealing with Customs paperwork and import duties and it is essential to make everything as easy as possible for them.

Shipping agents and express delivery companies are familiar with Incoterms and can provide account facilities to ensure agreed terms are complied with. With the appropriate authorisation, UPS for example can collect work from your studio and deliver it to a store in Japan, billing all transport and insurance costs to the buyer. When delivering work to a gallery in the USA, they can calculate the duty payable and either collect it from the customer or, if you quote prices 'Delivery Duty Paid', they will send you an invoice for it.

Remember that where your prices include import duty and taxes, you need to find out the rates applicable to your goods (according to the Customs classification code) from the commercial section of the embassy. Duty is payable on the invoice value of the goods plus the cost of freight and insurance.

Which currency?

It's hard enough negotiating prices in pounds without having to quote prices in different currencies. But it may be in your interest to offer that flexibility.

The basic rule is that when selling in this country, even to overseas buyers, deal in sterling. But if you are selling overseas, at a trade fair, market or exhibition, you will need to quote prices in the local currency. There are obvious exceptions: avoid accepting payment in a non-convertible currency or in the currency of a country subject

Susan Mason, *Vessel,* **pinched and coiled stoneware, 1993.**

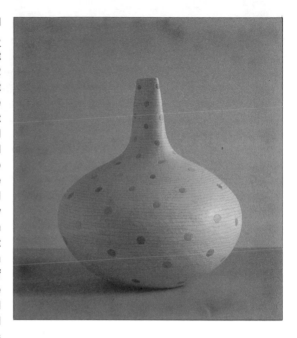

Susan Mason **has exhibited at the Messe Frankfurt in 1992 and 1993 through an East Midlands Arts initiative. The Messe, the world's largest trade show for fine craft and handmade gifts, has proved an excellent environment to promote Susan's work. She acknowledges her initial inexperience, showing only expensive one-off pieces in the first year which did not secure any orders. But in 1993 she presented a range of work, which included some less expensive jewellery and candlesticks, and returned with orders from across Europe, many for substantial amounts of work. She quotes prices in Deutschmarks and only takes proforma orders. She returns to Frankfurt in 1994, again part of a small group selected by East Midlands Arts who subsidise the cost of the stand to promote work from the region.**

to soaring inflation. And in these two situations, you should also be careful with the exchange rates used to work out payment in a more acceptable currency.

Makers have reported that American buyers often prefer dealing in dollars, even if they are in London for the Chelsea Craft Fair or in Germany for the Frankfurter Messe.

Export price lists

It rapidly becomes clear that you need separate price lists for overseas buyers which take account of the additional costs of exporting. Don't be tempted to over-inflate your prices for export. Some markets can bear it but, if anything, overseas buyers will be more price-conscious since they can order from anywhere in the world. The alternative to separate price lists is to spread the exporting costs across your existing prices but UK buyers may not accept the increases.

Nonetheless, in a situation where you are going to meet the market, as with an overseas trade fair, it is common practice to draw up price lists which take account of your expenses exhibiting there. If you are travelling to an overseas art or craft market or shipping your work for a selling exhibition, try to absorb the costs in your prices charged there. This means doing a rough calculation of how much you are likely to sell against the actual expenses incurred, eg transport, accommodation, show or market fees and insurance. With an overseas trade fair, you are likely to get more orders in the second and third years of attendance but try to keep your prices fairly consistent from one year to another by anticipating a lower level of orders at first.

When you quote prices in a foreign currency, it's important to cover yourself for any fluctuations in the exchange rate. Experienced exporters base their prices on the worst exchange rate option: a number of makers recommend allowing for around 25% fluctuation. For example, if the exchange rate is £1 = $1.40, use £1 = $1.75 (ie. $1.40 + 25%) as your base for converting prices into US dollars. This will avoid the need for frequent revisions of your foreign currency price lists. Don't print your special 'conversion rate' on the price list but keep a record of it on file. Buyers would not be impressed so keep quiet about it!

Taking orders

Taking an order or making an exhibition agreement with an overseas shop or gallery demands a greater degree of trust than within your own country. There may be a language barrier as well as different cultural and commercial practices. So it's important to retain that trust while safeguarding your professional interests.

Credit references

In America it is standard practice for a buyer to introduce themselves with a sheaf of credit referees and bank details. Elsewhere galleries and shops may not be so forthcoming but neither system can give you a cast iron guarantee. The best approach is to talk to other artists and makers with experience of that outlet. Talk to fellow trade fair or market exhibitors. Alternatively you could contact the national artists' or makers' association for that country. As well as a guarantee of the buyer's or gallery's trustworthiness, you want reassurance that the terms of trade offered (gallery commission rate, payment terms, etc) are acceptable practice.

When taking the first-time order from any overseas buyer, try to insist on proforma, although many major stores and museum shops are unlikely to agree to these terms. Proforma means receiving full payment in advance of dispatching the goods. It is normal to offer a discount of around 5% for proforma orders. If the customer agrees to place subsequent orders proforma, congratulations! But there are a range of acceptable alternatives. Sending the invoice at the same time as the goods with 30 days credit is normal international business practice. However, if the order is a large one, try negotiating a deposit. If the buyer won't agree, suggest dividing the order into smaller batches. If the customer knows a second batch won't arrive until payment is made for the first, they'll soon pay up.

Proforma pitfalls

Be aware that overseas buyers can be rather relaxed about proforma orders. Because the responsibility lies with them to make payment in advance of dispatch, you may find that some of these orders never materialise. An order with an agreed delivery date and 30 days credit is actually a firmer order than proforma, even though the payment is less guaranteed.

Jeweller Jane Adam finds that US buyers are very laid back about such things. She says they are delighted when you insist on proforma and often take it to mean that they only need decide if they really want the work when they return home. At a San Francisco trade fair, she found that around 25% of the proforma orders she took failed to materialise. Knowing this, she organises herself to make work only when the cheque arrives.

Neil Bottle has similar experience in a different selling situation. He reports that overseas buyers on a trip to Europe tend to start in London. He has an appointment to show them his work at an office or hotel and can come away with an 'order'. However, the buyers may be going on to Paris and Milan and only confirm orders once they return home. In his experience it can take up to six months for confirmation and orders may be consolidated up or down in quantity.

Getting paid

There are many different ways of paying for export orders including:
- cash
- cheque/Eurocheque (in sterling or foreign currency)
- credit card
- bank transfer
- cash on delivery to carrier
- letter of credit.

In order to decide which is best for you, first find out what your bank charges are for different types of foreign payment. Discuss it with the overseas department of your bank and get their advice.

If your agreement with the buyer is payment in advance of dispatch, always make sure the payment has cleared before you ship the goods. Your bank can advise you how long it takes for overseas cheque clearance.

Cheque

Surprisingly enough, it costs more to cash a sterling cheque from a foreign bank than one made out in a foreign currency. You could pay around £11-£17 to bank a sterling cheque drawn on a foreign bank whereas the charge for any number of foreign cheques in different currencies banked at the same time might be £6-£8. So it's not always a good idea to insist on payment in sterling from overseas customers unless they can produce a sterling cheque drawn on a UK bank.

Eurocheques can be a good way of accepting payment. They would be useful if you were selling work in a market since they are widely used in many European countries. A gallery or shop ordering work from you might also be able to pay by Eurocheque. When accepting payment look for the Eurocheque symbol on the cheque and guarantee card and verify the signature and account number. Eurocheques can be made out in the local currency or in sterling and the recipient pays no bank charges for payment in their own currency. Watch out for the cheque guarantee limit on Eurocheques. For sterling it is £100 but the limit is slightly different in other currencies. You can pay Eurocheques into a normal UK bank account and if you are travelling within Europe, ask your bank for details of how to open an account so that you can write cheques too.

Credit card

Where you are selling overseas, at a trade fair, market or on a selling trip to shops and galleries, it will be useful to have a credit card facility. Talk to your bank about getting a credit card facility. You will have to pay a percentage charge for every payment processed. Normally credit card facilities are restricted to UK sales in sterling only. So before you go, make sure you get authorisation from the credit card merchant section to accept payments abroad. The advantage of credit card is that the customer pays for any bank charges, ie currency conversion.

When you have a credit card facility, the bank issue you with the slide machine to imprint the customer's card. With the authorisation of the credit card company, it is generally acceptable to take the

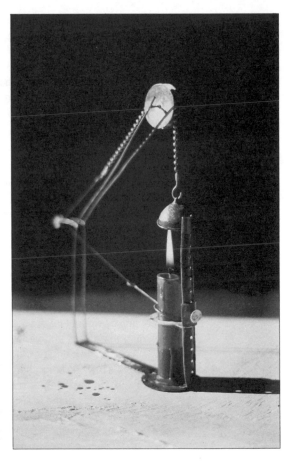

Jim Bond, *Dropper*, **copper and brass candle snuffer, 5" tall, 1992. Photo:** the artist

Jim Bond **makes automata and has developed a series of candle snuffing devices featuring magnetic spring and ballbearing extinguishing techniques. A Japanese gallery owner, visiting London, saw them in the Crafts Council's Victoria and Albert Museum shop and arranged to meet Jim. His introduction to exporting seems casual in contrast with others: "We met in a café in London, discussed the work and negotiated a price. She bought three candle snuffers to show in her Osaka gallery and paid in cash, passing me several hundred pounds under the table. I sent the work to Osaka by parcel post. It all arrived OK. We keep in touch as she comes to London on buying visits twice a year."**

machine abroad with you and accept payment from overseas customers but in sterling only. Access/Mastercard do open dollar accounts for some customers but only when there is a substantial volume of business. So accepting credit card payments abroad means converting prices back to sterling. And if your credit limit is low, it might mean making international telephone calls to get authorisation. Think it through and make sure you follow the correct procedures.

Bank transfer

Bank transfer is often one of the least expensive ways of getting paid. You need to supply your overseas customer with your bank name, address, name of the account, account number and sort code. They can then transfer money direct into your account. Find out whether the bank automatically sends out an advice when money is transferred in this way and check how long the transfer takes. SWIFT is a way of hastening money transfers through the international banking system. Any bank can advise on it.

Some banks offer special transfer facilities, often with cheaper charges. National Girobank operates an inexpensive and efficient direct electronic system which transfers funds in three days between customers in different countries who bank with the national post office bank. The Co-operative Bank is the UK representative for the Tipa-Net transfer system operating among co-operative banks in Belgium, France, Germany, Italy and Canada (America is due to join in 1994). Here the sender pays £5 and the recipient nothing. The money transfers within a week.

Cash on delivery
Parcelforce and a number of the express courier companies offer a CoD option on international deliveries. Obviously, you'll need to get the agreement of the person you are sending work to. Get the invoice to them well in advance of delivery, if necessary by fax. Before you agree this method of payment find out what the delivery company will charge for it (Parcelforce charges according to the amount to be collected, from £5 to £22.50) and how long it will take for them to pay the money over to you.

Letter of credit
See page 57, Example: 'Help! We're exporting and it's a nightmare'
This is a form of 'documentary credit' which is a special payment arrangement governed by an international commercial code. It is issued by the bank of the overseas buyer on their instruction and sent to the exporter's bank. Once you have received a copy from your bank the goods can be dispatched. The letter of credit guarantees that payment has been set aside by the buyer's bank and your bank collects it through the international bank transfer system.

Your bank will advise you when they have collected payment which can take around ten days. In order to release the money into your account, you need to present the bank with a series of documents: the commercial invoice, air waybill or consignment note, packing slips, declaration of country of origin and any other declarations required by the country of destination.

There are a number of different types of letter of credit, some more secure than others, so get advice from your bank. Also, before you agree to payment by letter of credit, find out what the charge will be. Textile designers Wallace Sewell found that letter of credit was the best method of payment on large US orders. However, it is does cost them £120 in bank charges per letter of credit. They are also obliged to give the customer a discount since it is considered a preferential method of payment for the supplier.

Overseas bank account

If you are doing regular business in one country, it may be a good idea to open a bank account there. As well as making it easier for payments, if you are spending time there on sales trips it will be convenient to have a local bank account. Make sure you understand how the account works and what charges will be levied. Don't assume that the bank account will work just as in Britain. UK customers, used to overdrafts and easy credit, can be shocked by the stricter banking codes in other countries where unauthorised overdrafts are treated almost as seriously as theft. In France the penalty for an unauthorised overdraft is withdrawal of your cheque book facility.

Chasing debts

Non-payment obviously causes more concern with an overseas customer. You certainly need to react quickly if an account becomes overdue. Contact the customer on a regular basis by post, fax, telephone or all three. Keep a record of when you call, who you speak to and what is said. Making overseas phone calls is expensive but necessary to chase unpaid bills. Experienced exporters anticipate this and build the cost into their prices.

If the invoice remains unpaid, you can hire a collection agency who will collect your debt for a fee. Jane Adam contacted an American collection agency who approached exhibitors at the New York Gift Fair. The service was quite straightforward. She handed over the unpaid invoice to the agency. Only if they managed to collect the money was a fee due (25% of the monies collected).

Export Credit Guarantees (ECG)

There is a Government-sponsored scheme which offers a form of insurance, known as ECGD cover, against non-payment of export orders. However, it is aimed at much larger businesses than most artists and makers are likely to operate. A credit insurance broker operating the scheme advised that it is only available for businesses with a minimum of £50,000 turnover per year in export business.

There are Export Credit Guarantee Departments covering all regions of the UK. The DTI can give you the address of the nearest office. However, they will probably refer you on to a broker dealing with small businesses. Alternatively, you can ask your bank, some of which provide export credit facilities. The system, known as factoring, means that as soon as goods are dispatched, the ECG insurance company pays you a large proportion of the invoice and takes the responsibly of collecting payment direct from the overseas company. They charge a percentage fee for the service.

VAT

See page 34, 'Customs and Excise' in 4 • Planning and preparation

VAT is a tax that only applies to countries in the European Union. It is imposed by EU legislation and is referred to as TVA in many of the other member states. It is a tax on sales of goods and services. At present, rates are not harmonised across the European Union although it is planned that eventually the rates and application of VAT will be the same in all member states.

In the UK, VAT at 17.5% is levied on sales of works of art created within the past 21 years and on many consumer goods. Only UK businesses with a turnover exceeding a certain threshold (£45,000 per year in 1994) are obliged to register and charge VAT although some business with a lower turnover may elect to do so. Therefore not many artists or makers are registered for VAT. In many other countries where VAT is in force, you'll find that most small businesses are registered as the threshold is much lower, as low as £7,000 in some countries.

Most exports by artists are zero rated for the purposes of VAT. This means that if you are registered, although you technically have to charge VAT on the sale, you do so at 0%, meaning that no VAT is actually added. In order to zero rate goods which are exported, different conditions apply depending on whether they are exported to the European Union or to a person outside those countries.

Trading outside the European Union
In order to zero rate goods exported outside the European Union you must have 'proof of export', eg a certificate of posting, air waybill or consignment note from a carrier. It is not acceptable for you to zero rate goods sold or delivered to any kind of intermediary who assures you that they will be exported, although they may subsequently zero rate them when they sell them on to someone outside the UK. Only delivery to a bona fide 'export packer', eg a freight carrier, courier firm or shipping company, is acceptable. If you cannot provide adequate proof of export, you become liable for VAT at the standard rate.

Trading within the European Union

For VAT-registered businesses trading in EU countries, there have been fundamental changes since January 1993. However, in spite of the desire to create an open market, it is astonishing how many impediments it has placed in the way of people trying to trade across the EU. It is actually now harder to trade in another European country than it was before the establishment of the Single European Market.

Trade within the EU is no longer described as import and export: movement of goods are now 'acquisitions' and 'supplies'. However, 'proof of export' is still required, as described above, to validate the zero rating of goods supplied to a customer in another EU country.

When you supply goods to a VAT-registered business in the European Union, it is necessary to show both your and their VAT number on the sales invoice. Both VAT numbers must include the country prefixes to identify them. If the customer is not registered for VAT and you are, you must charge the standard UK VAT rate on all sales to them.

If both you and the EU customer are VAT-registered, it is necessary to declare this fact on your VAT return. The net value of the goods supplied must be declared in box 8 of the return. In addition, you must prepare a European export sales listing. This is either prepared quarterly or, if you make prior application, annually. The annual return is only available to persons making relatively limited numbers of sales. This return must show for each return period the VAT number of the person you have exported to and the net value of the goods you have sold them. If this is not submitted on time a penalty can be imposed which can be at least £500 per late return. Customs and Excise documentation provides further information as to how to complete the returns.

Direct selling within the European Union

If you get involved in substantial levels of direct selling, VAT must also be considered. When you are selling to the public in another European Union country, either through direct selling or mail order, you are regarded as a trader there.

Special thresholds have been agreed for distance selling and if your turnover exceeds these you must register for VAT in that country. But the thresholds are quite high. For UK businesses, the current annual threshold for sales in France, Germany or the Netherlands is £70,000 and for sales in any other EU country it is £25,000. Below these thresholds, if you are a UK VAT-registered business, sales remain subject to UK VAT *unless* the customer can supply a VAT number for a European country.

There are special arrangements to ensure that UK Customs and Excise are aware of sales made where VAT is accounted for to another European Union country. Consult Customs and Excise on the matter should this situation arise.

Retail Export Scheme

If you are registered for VAT and find you sell work direct to individual customers from outside the European Union countries, it may be worthwhile offering those customers a VAT refund under the Retail Export Scheme. You are not obliged to offer this but it can secure a sale, especially with expensive work.

You decide whether you want to make an administration charge or set a minimum purchase level at which you will offer the scheme. An appropriate level would probably be at least £100 to justify a VAT refund. Even then, most of the refund would be taken up in bank charges paid by the customer.

The local Customs and Excise office can provide explanatory leaflets for the customer (VAT 704) and the Customs Form (VAT 407). Anyone proposing to use this scheme should obtain the latest documentation from Customs before doing so as the Retail Export Scheme does seem to change from time to time.

Currently a customer can only reclaim the VAT on goods to a maximum value of £600. Also goods purchased under the Retail Export Scheme must normally be carried through Customs in hand baggage. It is possible to reclaim the VAT on larger and heavier goods but the customer must contact the Customs export officer before they check in.

When a customer purchases work in the UK and plans to take it out of the country permanently, you complete the form VAT407 detailing goods purchased, your name and address and VAT number and the customer's name and home address. The customer always pays the VAT at the time of purchase. You must give them the Customs Form and a stamped self-addressed envelope for yourself. When they leave the country they take the form and goods to Customs at the airport for endorsement. Customs stamp the form which is then posted back to you in the envelope you provided. You then refund the VAT direct to the customer in whatever form you have agreed (eg International Money Order, sterling cheque).

Temporary exports

Many artists will occasionally export work to overseas galleries for exhibition and the work may be returned in due course. Arrangements for this vary slightly from country to country with regard to administrative detail.

The easiest arrangement for a VAT-registered UK artist exporting goods temporarily is to raise an invoice for Customs' purposes only. The invoice should show the VAT number of the gallery where the work is being sent. Then, subject to obtaining proof of export, the artist can zero rate the export and not pay VAT at that time. It would then be up to the gallery to work out the local arrangements for the payment of VAT, or not, on temporary import.

At the point the artist re-imports the work they must record that the goods have been brought back into the UK. This involves preparing a European acquisition listing for VAT purposes showing that the goods have been imported and their current value. This European acquisition listing must be retained. The artist then calculates the VAT at UK standard rate on this value, declares this sum as output VAT in box 2 of their VAT return and then adds an identical sum to their input VAT claim for the same quarter in box 4 of the VAT return. No VAT is actually paid to Customs and Excise on the re-import, just as none was paid on the export. But unless the proper declaration is made on the European acquisition listing and on the VAT return, a penalty can be imposed. These can be quite significant. Further clarification can be obtained from Customs and Excise.

Key points

- Selling work overseas takes more time and will incur additional expenses compared to selling work at home so it is important to plan for this and include the increased costs in your export prices.
- Be flexible about quoting your prices and accepting payment in other currencies.
- Getting paid is the main objective when you sell work abroad and there are many ways of accepting payment.
- Most exports by artists are zero rated for the purposes of VAT as long as certain conditions are met. The responsibility for providing incontrovertible proof of export lies with the registered business rather than the customer.
- VAT-registered traders who are unsure of how to deal with any import or export matter should always take specific advice from Customs and Excise prior to undertaking any transaction. Penalties for errors can be high and Customs have no sympathy with mistakes as they provide a free advice service for traders.

10 • Reviewing your progress

As an artist managing your own business or independent practice, it is vital to make time to stand back and review your progress. It may be that you started exporting by chance. Or perhaps you approach selling and exhibiting abroad as part of a planned strategy. Either way, it is important to look at what you have achieved, acknowledge your successes and plan the way forward.

When to review

Your exporting activities are an integral part of your work and life as an artist so try not to view them in isolation. An annual review is a good idea and should be combined with an overview of everything else you are doing.

Choose a time of the year when you are not too busy and can approach the review in an optimistic frame of mind. Just after New Year suits some while for others, spring or autumn might be the season for looking forward when you naturally devote time and energy to planning for the future. If you want to focus on the financial rewards of export sales, plan your review to coincide with completing your annual accounts.

Information gathering

Your first task is to gather the details of all your exporting activities during the past year. What you choose to include depends on how you define 'exporting' for yourself. Whatever your field of interest, include both action (eg sales and exhibitions) and research into overseas opportunities. Look at the following questions:

- Which countries have you sold or exhibited in?

• Who are your customers and exhibition contacts?

• Where have you found them or how have they found you?

• What is your income from export sales?

• What percentage of your turnover does it represent?

• What research have you undertaken?

• What problems have you encountered?

• Which areas (geographical or other) would you like to develop?

Next it's important to analyse the information and devise a plan for the coming year. There are various techniques for doing this.

SWOT analysis

Many makers and artists who have had some business enterprise training are familiar with the SWOT analysis. This consists of appraising your current position by assessing the Strengths and Weaknesses you and your work bring and the Opportunities and Threats posed by the environment you work in.

It is a useful exercise which can really help in decision-making so it's worth spending some time doing it. You can take a broad theme such as 'Exporting my work' or 'Developing opportunities abroad' or you may want help in deciding between two possible courses of action, eg 'Exhibiting at XYZ trade show in America' or 'Going on a marketing trip to galleries in Germany and the Netherlands'. In the latter case you will need to do a separate SWOT for each course of action and compare the two.

You'll end up with a fairly long list under each of the four headings (internal Strengths and Weaknesses and external Opportunities and Threats). The value of the SWOT analysis is in how you use that information to plan for the future. Sometimes the results indicate a clear way forward, sometimes not, but it can help you feel more confident about the things you are doing well and make informed decisions about the areas where you would benefit from advice, information or training.

Mind mapping

Some of the business review methods are too rational and analytical to help artists in their decision-making. Creative minds are often more at ease with 'right brain' techniques such as mind-mapping.

Take a large sheet of paper and write in the centre 'Exporting', 'Exhibiting abroad' or whatever you want to explore. Next you write down all your activities relating to this, arranged around the centre.

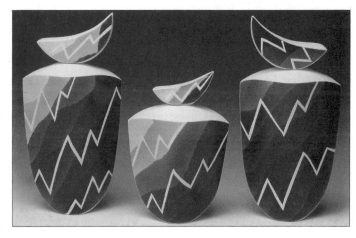

Sasha Wardell, slip-cast bone china with airbrushed decoration, 19cm high.

Sasha Wardell took a radical approach to exporting. She moved to France in 1989. She has continued to sell and exhibit her work, widening her network in mainland Europe. Two agents promote her work to shops and galleries in Benelux, Germany and Switzerland. Recent exhibitions include shows in Brussels, Holland, Barcelona and Hamburg. Paradoxically her work is less well recognised in France where there is less familiarity with slip-cast work used in a contemporary context. But working in France has brought new opportunities and she now runs specialised courses in bone china techniques with trainees from across Europe and as far afield as India, Taiwan and Africa.

Use different coloured pens to represent types of work, geographical areas or good and bad experiences. A pattern will emerge, with your exporting experiences radiating out from the centre like spokes on a wheel. Some activities will be closer to the centre than others. Link them up where appropriate so that you can see where one action has led to many more contacts and projects and where another has been a dead end. The good experiences will stand out as colourful, bold and decorated while the bad ones will look plain and black.

Mind mapping helps you see the patterns in your actions. Using this technique can help you decide where to invest your efforts in the future. It can help you pinpoint areas of uncertainty such as the tensions caused by that exciting trip to a trade show in San Francisco where your work got a great reception but the downside was that it was very expensive and involved spending too much time away from your family.

Getting advice

One conclusion from the review might be that you need some business advice. If you are under 26 you can get free advice through the Livewire network. Up to 29 years you can turn to the Prince's Youth Business Trust who offer grants and free business advice. Whatever your age, specialist paid consultations on exporting can be arranged through the DTI (usually with your local Chamber of Commerce) who have appointed Export Development Advisors around the country.

Moving forward

A longer-term strategy for exporting will help you build on your successes and make sound decisions on where best to invest for the future.

First you need to clarify your objectives. This means re-stating why you want to promote yourself and your work overseas. Artists' and makers' priorities vary enormously, eg to make a living; to gain an international reputation; for the stimulus of new places, people, languages and challenges; to connect with cultural roots; to work in a way not possible in the UK; to network with artists in other countries.

A longer-term strategy places your main objectives at its heart. Decide what proportion of your time you can devote to furthering these objectives and plan accordingly. Write down all the things you'd like to do in the next year to develop overseas opportunities. Make them as specific as possible, eg 'Enter my work in five open exhibitions or competitions in Europe' rather than 'Have some exhibitions abroad'. Check whether your action list is realistic and achievable and allocate extra time to respond to unexpected opportunities.

Build on your contacts

Whether you are building up business through export sales or developing opportunities by networking with artists abroad, one strong principle holds. Always try to build on existing contacts rather than dissipating your energy in endlessly chasing more.

It's easy to become boggled by all the information available. But one solid achievement, however small, is worth more than an address book full of world-wide artists' contacts. You will gain more success and satisfaction by investing yourself fully in one market, project or area of work than by spreading your efforts thinly across them all. A commitment to a particular country might mean learning the language or studying the culture.

Persistence, together with the quality of your follow-up, are the key to developing a solid international reputation. Whether you are showing at a New York trade show or demonstrating ceramics techniques in Australia, the second time you visit will always be more rewarding. You're already known there and because you know what to expect, you are better prepared. By the third and fourth trips, you can relax and enjoy the ease with which you deal with previously unfamiliar situations. Your contacts in the country have become real friends.

Then you can appreciate just how far you've progressed from when you viewed exporting as a series of problems to be solved. Working internationally has become a way of life.

Key points

- By reviewing your progress on a regular basis you can make sound decisions on where you want to invest your effort over the next year.
- You need to consider your exporting activities as an integral part of your business or independent practice as an artist.
- Start the review by gathering the information on your international activities over the past year.
- The SWOT analysis or mind-mapping techniques can help you analyse that information in a way which helps you plan for the future.
- A long-term strategy for exporting involves building up your contacts and concentrating your efforts on a small number of markets, perhaps just one country. A deeper understanding of the people, culture and networks in just a few places will ultimately be more rewarding, both in terms of business and personal satisfaction.

11 • Glossary

Air Waybill The 'contract of carriage' for goods shipped by air. This document is given to you by the freight company. It should be retained as it acts as proof of export.

Bill of lading The 'contract of carriage' for goods shipped by sea. It acts as proof of export and as title to ownership of the goods. The document must be transferred to the overseas customer to enable them to claim the goods.

British returned goods Goods exported but subsequently returned to the UK. This wording should be used on any consignment of goods returned in these circumstances. When you produce proof of export (the contract of carriage document), goods will be released by UK Customs without any duty payable.

C&F Cost and freight (see under Incoterms).

Carnet Also known as ATA Carnet. ATA stands for 'Admission Temporaire – Temporary Admission'. The Carnets are multi-sheet documents issued by Chambers of Commerce, with the backing of a bank guarantee. They are used for the temporary export and re-import of goods, eg for an exhibition.

CIF Cost, insurance and freight (see under Incoterms).

Collection agency Company which collects unpaid debts against a percentage fee of the amount collected.

Commercial invoice A document, required for all goods being exported, which you produce on your own headed paper. It gives precise details of the goods to be exported and their destination. See Chapter 8 for information to be included.

Commodity code See Tariff number.

Consignment note The 'contract of carriage' for goods transported by road. The document is issued by the freight company and should be retained as it acts as proof of export.

Contract of carriage A document issued by the freight company shipping goods overseas which acts as proof of export. Depending on means of transport used, it may be the air waybill, bill of lading or consignment note.

Declarations Official statements required for goods exported to certain countries, eg Declaration of Country of Origin (required by most countries). See the relevant country section in *Croner's Reference Book for Exporters* for any special declarations required.

Delivery Duty Paid (see under Incoterms).

Documentation Paperwork required by Customs for exporting goods.

DTI Department of Trade and Industry. The government department responsible for exporting. Practical help, advice and support available through the Overseas Trade Services network.

Duty Payment collected by Customs and Excise of the receiving country where goods are imported. Each country's government sets its own rates of duty with different percentages according to type of goods.

EFTA European Free Trade Association (Austria, Switzerland, Sweden, Norway, Finland, Iceland and Liechtenstein). Countries which have established preferential trade agreements with EU countries.

EU European Union (formerly known as the European Community/EC). Includes the UK, Republic of Ireland, France, Germany, Belgium, Luxembourg, Netherlands, Denmark, Spain, Italy, Portugal and Greece.

ExWorks / ExFactory (see under Incoterms).

Export credit guarantees A system for insuring payments for exported goods. Credit insurance is administered by the government's Export Credit Guarantee Department and is offered by certain banks and through specialised insurance brokers. Generally only appropriate for businesses with an export turnover in excess of £50,000 per year.

Export Licence An export licence is required for valuable objects and works of art at least 50 years old. Export licences are issued by the Department of National Heritage.

Factoring A scheme offered by credit insurance companies to businesses with a high turnover in export sales. They 'factor' your invoices for a fee by paying you as soon as goods are shipped and taking responsibility for collecting payment from the overseas customer.

FOB Free on board (see under Incoterms).

Freight General term for transport of goods overseas, eg air freight, road freight.

Harmonised System An internationally recognised system, operated in almost every country, for coding goods in transit. Tariff numbers can be obtained by consulting the *HM Customs & Excise Tariff* in a public library.

Incoterms

C&F Cost and freight. The price of the goods includes freight charges to a named port of destination, paid by the exporter, but excluding the cost of insurance.

CIF Cost, insurance, freight. The price for goods delivered to a named port of destination, with the exporter paying freight and insurance charges on the goods up to that point.

Delivery Duty Paid Price includes transport, insurance and any duty and taxes payable, delivered to the customer.

ExWorks (or ExFactory) The basic price as if goods were collected from your place of work.

FOB Free on board. The price at which goods are delivered on board the vessel with transport to this point at the exporter's expense.

LEC Local Enterprise Council (Scottish equivalent to TEC – see below).

Letter of credit A type of documentary credit which ensures payment for exported goods is collected through the international banking system. Requires meticulous attention to export paperwork since payment is only released by your bank on sight of relevant documents. Incurs substantial bank charges.

Packing slip Document often required for export detailing goods contained in each package of a consignment. The packing slip should be attached to the package. Keep two copies.

Proforma Type of invoice giving details of goods or services to be supplied when payment is received. It secures payment in advance of dispatch of goods.

Proof of export Document (usually the contract of carriage) which proves goods have been exported.

Retail Export Scheme System which allows you to offer overseas customers (living outside the European Union) purchasing work direct from you in the UK to obtain a refund on the VAT. For VAT-registered businesses only. Contact the VAT office for forms.

SAD (Single Administrative Document) Document issued by Customs and Excise for export of goods. Get advice from a shipping agent on where this is required.

Shipping General term normally used for transporting goods abroad. Any form of transport may be used, road, rail and air as well as sea.

Tariff number Also known as the commodity code. Multi-digit number which identifies goods transported. Tariff numbers are determined by the Harmonised System, an internationally recognised system.

TECs Training and Enterprise Councils, called LECs in Scotland. Agencies which administer Enterprise Allowance scheme and offer business counselling and training advice.

SOME USEFUL VOCABULARY

This brief section includes some of the terms which are particularly prone to mistranslation. Unless you are fluent, always engage a professional translator with a specialised knowledge of technical terms to produce a statement about your work in another language.

Key: French (Fr), German (Ge), American (US).

Art form *Discipline* (Fr), *Sparte* (Ge).

Artists' workshop There is a strong tradition of residential workshops for artists in many other countries. 'Plener' or 'symposium' are terms used in Central and Eastern Europe. In the United States, they may be described as 'artists' colonies'.

Application form *Dossier d'inscription* (Fr).

Craft *Artisanat d'art* (Fr), *Kunsthandwerk* (Ge).

CV *Curriculum* (Fr), *Resumé* (US).

Education/Training *Formation* (Fr), *Ausbildung* (Ge).

Exhibition *Exposition* (Fr), *Ausstellung* (Ge).

Grants/Scholarships *Bourses* (Fr), *Stipendien* (Ge).

Jewellery *Bijouterie* (Fr), *Schmuck* (Ge).

Placement/Residency *Internship* (US).

Potter *Töpfer* (Ge).

SAE *SASE* (US).

Slide *Diapositive* (Fr), *Dia* (Ge).

Submission fee *Droit de présentation* (Fr), *Teilnahmgebühr* (Ge).

Visual arts *Arts plastiques* (Fr). Often mistranslated from French and other latin languages as 'plastic arts'. Artists are *plasticiens* (Fr).

Work (of art) *Oeuvre* (Fr), *Arbeit/Werk* (Ge).

12 • Contacts

Councils and boards

Arts Council of England, 14 Great Peter Street, London, SW1P 3NQ, tel: 0171 333 0100. Only funds projects and programmes of 'national significance' including research and touring exhibitions. Other funding undertaken in England by the regional arts boards see below.

Arts Council of Northern Ireland, 185 Stranmillis Road, Belfast, BT9 5DU, tel: 01232 381 591. Funded by the Office of Northern Ireland.

Arts Council of Wales, Museum Place, Cardiff, CF1 3NX, tel: 01222 394711. Covers visual arts and crafts in Wales.

Crafts Council, 44a Pentonville Road, London, N1 9HF, tel: 0171 278 7700. Provides setting up grants for individuals, subsidy for touring exhibitions. Comprehensive information service available by letter, telephone or in person.

East Midlands Arts Board, Mountfields HouseForest Road, Loughborough, LE11 3HU, tel: 01509 218292. Covers Leicestershire, Nottinghamshire, Northamptonshire and Derbyshire except High Peak District.

Eastern Arts Board, Cherry Hinton Hall, Cherry Hinton Road, Cambridge, CB1 4DW, tel: 01223 215355. Covers Bedfordshire, Cambridge, Essex, Hertfordshire, Lincolnshire, Norfolk, Suffolk.

London Arts Board, Elme House, 133 Long Acre, London, WC2E 9AF, tel: 0171 240 1313. Covers Greater London.

North West Arts Board, 4th Floor, 12 Harter Street, Manchester, M1 6HY, tel: 0161 228 3062. Covers Cheshire, Greater Manchester, Lancashire, Merseyside and High Peak District of Derbyshire.

Northern Arts Board, 9/10 Osborne Terrace, Newcastle upon Tyne, NE2 1NZ, tel: 0191 281 6334. Covers Cleveland, Cumbria, Durham, Northumberland, and Tyne & Wear.

Scottish Arts Council, 12 Manor Place, Edinburgh, EH3 7DO, tel: 0131 226 6051. Covers visual arts and crafts in Scotland.

South East Arts Board, 10 Mount Ephraim, Tunbridge Wells, TN4 8AS, tel: 01892 515210. Covers Kent, Surrey and East & West Sussex, excluding Greater London areas.

South West Arts Board, Bradninch PlaceGandy Street, Exeter, EX4 3LS, tel: 01392 218188. Covers Avon, Cornwall, Devon and Dorset, except Bournemouth, Christchurch and Poole areas, Gloucestershire and Somerset.

Southern Arts Board, 13 St Clements Street, Winchester, SO23 9UQ, tel: 01962 55099. Covers Berkshire, Buckinghamshire, Hampshire, Isle of Wight, Oxfordshire, Wiltshire, and the Poole, Bournemouth and Christchurch areas of Dorset.

West Midlands Arts Board, 82 Granville Street, Birmingham, B1 2LH, tel: 0121 631 3121. Covers Hereford & Worcester, Shropshire, Staffordshire, Warwickshire and West Midlands.

Yorkshire and Humberside Arts Board, 21 Bond Street, Dewsbury, WF13 1AX, tel: 01924 455555. Covers Humberside and North, South & West Yorkshire.

Export buying houses

Note: inclusion in this list does not constitute a recommendation

AGAL, 9 Frederick Mews, Kinnerton St, London SW1X 8EQ, tel: 0171 823 2660. Represent major department stores in the USA (Bergdorf Goodman, Neimann Marcus) and the Far East.

British Isles Buying Agency, 7-11 Lexington St, London W1R 3HQ, tel: 0171 494 2151. Represent stores across the USA.

EXBO Export Buying Offices Association, Londwood, Cadogan Pier, Chelsea Embankment, London SW3 5RQ, fax: 0171 351 9287.

Association of London buying offices with members representing major department stores in the USA, Australia, Japan, Singapore, Taipei and Hong Kong.

Isetan, 28 Bruton St, London W1X 7DB, tel: 0171 495 0003. Represent Isetan stores in the Far East (Japan, Singapore, Hong Kong).

Takashimaya (UK) Ltd, Brook Street House, 47 Davies St, London W1Y 1FJ, tel: 0171 493 3312. Represents Takashimaya department stores in Japan, Singapore, New York, Taipei and Sydney.

Express delivery services

Note: inclusion in this list does not constitute a recommendation

DHL, Orbital Park, 178-188 Great South West Road, Hounslow, Middlesex TW4 6JS, tel: 01345 100300 (local rate). Delivery to 270 countries worldwide.

Federal Express, Federal Express House, Bond Gate, Nuneaton, Warks CV11 4AI, tel: 0800 123800 (freephone). Delivery to North and South America, Middle and Far East, Australasia. Not Europe.

Parcelforce International, tel: 0800 224466 (freephone). Delivery worldwide.

Securicor Omega Express: Network Europe, Ponton Road, London SW8 5BA, tel: 01345 200345 (local rate). Delivery to European Union, Switzerland and Scandinavia.

TNT, 161-163 Staines Road, Hounslow, Middx TW3 3JB, tel: 0800 776000 (freephone). Delivery to most countries worldwide.

UPS United Parcel Service, UPS House, Forest Road, Feltham, Middx TW13 7DY, tel: 0800 456789 (freephone). Worldwide Express delivery to over 180 countries, Euro Express delivery service to all European countries.

Grants and advice

British Council, Visual Arts Department11 Portland Place, London, W1N 4EJ, tel: 0171 930 8406. Provides contact with 90 countries through 162 offices abroad where funds may be available to assist in-coming artists. May provide some help to artists with firm invitations to exhibit abroad. Leaflet Studying Abroad (from Education Information Centre, 10 Spring Gardens, London SW1A 2BN), briefly describes schemes they administer.

Calouste Gulbenkian Foundation, 98 Portland Place, London, W1N 4ET, tel: 0171 636 5313, fax: 0171 636 2948. New Horizons Artist's Bursaries, offered in 1992 and 1993, are designed to help experienced artists (writers, performing, media and visual artists) work in a new art form.

Central Bureau for Educational Visits and Exchanges, Seymour Mews House, Seymour Mews, London, W1H 9PE, tel: 0171 486 5101, fax: 0171 935 5741. Grant and bursary schemes to encourage study abroad and co-operation in education. Young Workers Exchange Programme and Youth for Europe also organised.

Commonwealth Foundation Fellowships, Education Division, Commonwealth Institute, Kensington High St, London, W8 6NQ, tel: 0171 603 4535 ext 300, fax: 0171 602 7374. Information and awards for study at universities in Commonwealth countries.

David Canter Memorial Trust, PO Box 3, Ashburton, Devon, TQ13 7UW. Annual awards to makers for travel or special projects.

Erasmus, 15 rue d'Arlon, 1040 Brussels, Belgium, tel: [00 32] 2 233 0111. Grants for academic staff to undertake temporary teaching assignments in EC universities including travel grants for making contacts in other countries. Exchanges of between 3 months and a year.

European Pepinieres for Young People, 6 rue de Braque, 75003 Paris, France, tel: [00 33] 44 54 36 30, fax: [00 33] 44 54 36 31, contact: Pierre Keryvin. Biennially offers 3-6 month residencies with workspace, accommodation and living expenses to artists in various artistic disciplines in European cities. Short-list decided by national panel, final candidates by international jury.

Foundation for Sport and the Arts, PO Box 20, Liverpool, L9 6EA, tel: 0151 524 0235, contact: 051 524 0285. Offers support to individual artists based on project proposals.

Fulbright Fellowships, UK Educational Commission, 6 Porter St, London, W1M 2HR, tel: 0171 486 7697, fax: 0171 224 4567. Annual award for an artist to spend six months in the US, and other awards to encourage direct exchange of US/UK teaching posts. Postgraduate and student travel awards also made annually. Details published annually in Artists Newsletter.

German Academic Exchange Service (DAAD), 2 Bloomsbury Square, London, WC1A 2LP, tel: 0171 404 4065. Offers study visits, scholarships and research grants in various categories.

Kaleidoscope, Commission of the European Communities, UK Office, 8 Storey's Gate, London, SW1P 3AT. Annual awards with changing categories covering all artforms to support cultural events which involve at least three European partners. Deadline for 1994 was 1 December 1993.

Kathleen and Margery Flint Scholarships, 10 Bennett Hill, Birmingham, B2 5RS. Educational exchange grants including maintenance and travel for projects which have already gained some funding.

LEDU, LEDU House, Upper Galwally, Belfast, BT8 4TB, tel: 01232 491031. Provides advice and training for small businesses in N Ireland.

Leverhulme Trust, Lintas House, New Fetter Lane, London, EC4, tel: 0171 822 5252. Gives awards anually, some for travel.

Portugal 600, Palingswick House241 King Street, London, W6 9LP. Go and See grants for UK/ Republic of ireland residents aged 26 or over or young people 18-26 not in full-time eduction. Maximum £500.

Prince's Trust, 8 Bedford Row, London, WC1R 4BA, tel: 0171 405 5799, contact: Anne Engel. Offers schemes which assist young people (under 25, or under 29 if disabled) to make contacts in Europe including Richard Mills Travel Fellowships, Go and See, Go Ahead and European Vision.

Prince's Youth Business Trust, 5th Floor, 5 Cleveland Place, London, SW1Y 6JJ, tel: 0171 321 6500, fax: 0171 834 6494. Helps designers and artists between the ages of 18-29 to set up in business, providing financial advice and grants and loans of up to £5000.

Rome Scholarships, British School at Rome, Tuke Building, Regents College, Inner Circle, Regents Park, London, 0171 487 7403. Offers accommodation, studio and subsistence for UK artists to work and study in Rome. Details published annually in Artists Newsletter.

Training and Enterprise Councils (TECs). See telephone directory for local details. Advice, information and training on a business set-up and development, including exporting. For Scotland, contact Local Enterprise Councils and Northern Ireland, Local Enterprise Development Unit.

Winston Churchill Memorial Trust, 15 Queensgate Terrace, London, SW7 5PR, tel: 0171 584 9315. Has annual travel award but applications need to take notice of the fact that catagories are rarely art specific – eg 'environment'. Details published annually in Artists Newsletter.

Information

Association of British Chambers of Commerce, 9 Tufton Street, London, SW1P 3QB, tel: 0171 222 1555. Contact for the Chamber of Commerce in your area, but see also 'Yellow Pages'.

Association of Commonwealth Universities, John Foster House, 36 Gordon Square, London, WC1H 0PF, tel: 0171 387 8572. Offers a publication and information service through small reference library (appointment necessary); can offer advice on awards, fellowships and scholarships.

British American Arts Association, 116 Commercial Street, London, E1 6NF, tel: 0171 247 5385. Information resource to aid professional artists to work in US and develop links and exchanges in Europe. Reference library open to personal callers.`

British Exporters Association, 16 Dartmouth St, London SW1H 9BL, tel: 0171 222 5419

British Standards Institution, Linford Wood, Milton Keynes, MK14 6LE, tel: 01908 220022. Technical help to exporters.

Centre for European Business Information, Small Firms Service, 11 Belgrave Road, London, SW1V 1RB, tel: 0171 828 6201. Free information pack and details of other centres.

Commission of the European Union, Jean Monnet House, 8 Storey's Gate, London, SW1P 3AT, tel: 0171 973 1992, fax: 0171 973 1900. Information service including details of institutions, study and courses in EU countries open to visitors between 10-1pm daily and for telephone queries 2-5pm.

Design & Artists Copyright Society Ltd (DACS), St Mary's Clergy House, 2 Whitechurch Lane, London, E1 7QR, tel: 0171 247 1650. Covers visual artists including photographers and art video-makers and protects members' copyright interests. Agreements with 23 societies worldwide who provide reciprocal services.

DTI (Department of Trade & Industry), tel: 0181 200 1992. Provides information to help British businesses compete in UK, Europe and elsewhere. Regional offices: N East 0191 232 4722; N West 0161 838 5228 & 0151 227 4111; Yorks & Humbs 0113 244 3171; E Midlands 0115 950 6181; W Midlands 0121 212 5000; East 01223 461939; S West 0117 927 2666; S East 0171 215 0574, 01737 226900, 0734 395600; Wales 01222 825111; Scotland 0141 248 2855; N Ireland 01232 233 3233.

DTI Export Market Information Centre (EMIC), Ashdown House 123 Victoria Street, London, SW1E 6RB, England, tel: 0171 2155444. Extensive library with market research information

European Commission, Jean Monnet House, 8 Storey's Gate, London SW1P 3AT, tel: 0171 973 1992, fax: (Information Services Unit) 0171 973 1900. Note: there can be a long queue for information so faxing enquiries in worth doing.

European Documentation Centres. 45 UK Regional centres which house EU databases on legislation, directives, standards, statistics, etc. For the address of your nearest EDC contact the European Commission office (above).

Euro Information Centres, Information on legislation, EU research/development programmes, law, grants/loans, etc; contacts, trade fairs, etc. Belfast 01232 491031; Birmingham 0121 454 6171; Bradford 01274 752462; Brighton 01273 220870; Bristol 0117 973 7373; Cardiff 01222 229525; Exeter 01392 214085; Glasgow 0141 221 0999; Inverness 01464 234121; Leeds 0113 243 9222; Leicester 0116 255 4464; Liverpool 0151 298 1928; London 0171 261 1163/ 489 1992; Maidstone 01622 694109; Manchester 0161 236 3210; Newcastle 0191 261 0026; Norwich 01603 625977; Nottingham 0115 962 4624; Slough 01753 577 8777; Telford 01952 588766; Southampton 01703 832866; Stafford 01785 59528.

Euro-Link for Lawyers, tel: 0113 242 2845. Networking association which can put you in touch with a lawyer specialising in any field of law in any community country or city for whose advice you then pay.

Eurodesk. Provides information on training, education and youth activities in the EU by subscription. **Eurodesk Central Bureau**, Seymour Mews House, Seymour Mews, London, W1H 9PE, tel: 0171 4865101. **Eurodesk European centre**, Paradise Road, Plymouth, PL1 5QL, tel: 01752 385353. **Eurodesk Scottish Community Education Council**, Rosebery House 9 Haymarket Terrace, Edinburgh, EH12 5EZ, tel: 0131 3132488. **EuroEd Wales**, Orchard House Orchard Street, Swansea, SA1 5DJ, tel: 01792 457456.

HM Customs & Excise, New Kings Beam House, 22 Upper Ground, London SE1 9PJ, tel: 0171 620 1313 (Head Office).

National Artists Association (NAA), Spitalfields, 21 Steward Street, London E1 6AJ, tel 0171 426 0911. Representative body for visual artists. Offers advice and information through conferences, publications and other activities. Involved with establishing professional qualifications for artists, and with protection of artists' rights in collaboration with other organisations. Member of European Artists Council.

One Stop Shops. Contact your local TEC to see whether a one stop shop has been set up in your area.

PETRA, Central Bureau of Educational Visits and Exchanges, Seymour Mews, London, W1H 9PE, tel: 0171 486 5101, fax: 0171 935 5741. Aims to raise standards and the quality of technical and vocational education, stimulate trans-national co-operations and partnerships and promote European training. Encourages exchanges and work placements in Europe for young people.

Transport Firms

Note: inclusion in this list does not constitute a recommendation.

C'Art, 48 Paget Road, Wolverhampton, tel: 01902 26073. Art and craft transport throughout Britain and Europe.

Artlink Transport, 102 Main Street, Milngavie, Glasgow, tel: 0141 956 5320.

James Bourlet, 3 Space Way, Feltham, Feltham, TW14 OTY, tel: 0181 751 1155.

Matt Cranmer, tel: 0181 318 2448.

Rees Martin Art Service, Unit 3129-131 Coldharbour Lane, London, SE5 9NY, tel: 0171 274 5555. Transport

Securicor Omega Express, Network Europe, Ponton Road, London, SW8 5BA, tel: 01345 200345. Delivery to European Union, Switzerland and Scandinavia

Shuttle Services, Roy Eadon, tel: 0191 281 1397

Transnic Ltd, Arch 434, Gordon Grove, London, SE5 9DU, tel: 0171 738 7555.

13 • Further reading

AA Astro Artz and Fringe

Available from: Fringe Festival Los Angeles, 6380 Wilshire Blvd., Suite 147, Los Angeles, CA 90048, USA.

Doing it right in LA: Self producing for the performing artist, Jacki Apple, 1990, ISBN 0 937122 13 0. Resource book for performing artists covering choosing the site, budgeting, selecting performers, finding materials, publicity and promotion and the performance itself. Price: $12.00 exc p&p.

AFAA

Available from AFAA, 45 rue Boissière, 75116 Paris, France. Few remaining copies in stock, no current plans to reprint. Price: 120FF ex p&p.

L'Accueil d'artistes en résidence temporaire en France (Guide of host facilities for artists on short-term stay in France), AFAA, March 1992. Very useful and detailed bilingual guide produced by French Ministry of Culture.

AN Publications

Available from: AN Publications, PO Box 23, Sunderland SR4 6DG tel 0191 514 3600. Post £1.50 per order.

Across Europe – the artist's personal guide to travel and work, 1st edition, ed. David Butler, 1992, ISBN 0 907730 15 9. Artists' experiences of exhibiting, living and working in 24 European countries with lists of contacts, resources and background information on each country. Price: £9.95.

Artists Newsletter. Monthly magazine for artists, makers and photographers, lists commissions and other opportunities in the UK and abroad with news about a range of completed visual arts and crafts projects and practical and discursive articles. Price: £19.95 UK annual subscription 12 issues.

Fact Pack: Artists and the EU, Emma Lister, 1993. Contact list for countries in the European Union Price: £1.85 inc p&p.

Fact Pack: Craft Fairs, Kathryn Salomon, 1991. Including a selected list of those held national and (a few) internationally. Updated annually Price: £1.85 inc p&p.

Fact Pack: Slide Indexes, 1993. Listing 40 indexes and registers in the UK, with details of eligibility and who consults them. Some indexes will be consulted by visitors from abroad. Price: £1.85 inc p&p.

Fundraising: the artist's guide to planning and financing work, ed. Susan Jones, 1993, ISBN 0 907730 20 5. Drawing on artists' experiences and advice, demonstrates the many ways artists and groups can finance exhibitions, travel, projects etc ranging from grants from arts boards and trusts to loans and sponsorship. Includes advice on writing applications, matching funding and budgeting Price: £7.25 inc p&p.

Introduction to Contracts, Nicholas Sharp, 1993. Outlines elements and terms in legal contracts, with advice on how to negotiate, deal with disputes and find a solicitor. Price: £1.50 inc p&p.

Licensing Reproductions, Nicholas Sharp, 1994. Explains in straightforward terms how to grant or obtain permission to reproduce artwork or designs. Includes sample licence and royalty agreements that can be photocopied for personal use. Advice on types of agreements, fees and royalties, negotiating and monitoring agreements Price: £3.50 inc p&p.

Making Ways: the visual artist's guide to surviving and thriving, 3rd edition, ed. David Butler, 1992, ISBN 0 907 730 16 7. Covers exhibiting, selling, working in public and with people, collective action, skill sharing, publicity and promotion, studios, health and safety, employment and legal issues, insurance, contracts and copyright with reading and contacts lists. Price: £11.99.

Money Matters, 2nd edition, Sarah Deeks, Richard Murphy & Sally Nolan, 1991, ISBN 0 907730 26 4. Artist's financial guide to self-employment covering taxation, VAT, NIC. Includes accounting system devised especially for artists and makers. Price: £7.25.

Organising Your Exhibition – the self-help guide, 2nd edition, Debbie Duffin, ISBN 0 907730 14 0. Covering finding space, finance, timetabling, publicity, promotion, framing, security and insurance, transporting work, hanging, private view, selling work and making the best of an exhibition. Price: £7.25.

Selling, Judith Staines, 1993, ISBN 0 907730 19 1. Practical advice, based on artists' experiences, of promoting and selling art and craft work. Price: £7.25.

Selling Contracts, Nicholas Sharp, 1993. Includes four model contracts, which can be photocopied for personal use, covering direct sales of art and craft work to private buyers, galleries and shops, and sale or return agreements Price: £3.50 inc p&p.

Arts Council of England

Available from: Arts Council of England, 14 Great Peter Street, London SW1P 3NQ

An Introductory Guide to Travel Opportunities for Black Art Practitioners, Susan Okokon, 1991. Lists organisations, trusts and educational opportunities, although as it was produced in 1991, some information is now out-of-date. Price: £5 inc p&p.

Arts Networking in Europe, Rod Fisher, 1992. Contact names, addresses and information of more than 140 European arts networks including some relevant to visual arts. Price: £10 inc p&p.

On the Road: the start-up guide to touring the arts in Europe, July 1993. Price £10 inc p&p.

Women in Arts: creating networks, ed Alex Ankrah, 1993, ISBN 0 728706 79 2. International directory of women working in the arts. Price £4 inc p&p.

Arts Council of Ireland

Available from: Available from AN Publications (see above)

Handle with Care, ed. John Hunt. Guidance on the care and handling of artworks and exhibitions. Chapters on packing, transport and export of artworks. Price: £5 inc p&p.

Associated Management Services

Available from: Associated Management Services, Grant Guide Department, 10 Broad Street, Swindon, Wilts SN1 2DR.

Guide to Grants for Business, 5nd edition, 1993. Covers UK Government grants and loans, European Union grants and includes local contacts. Price £39.50.

British American Arts Association

Available from: 116 Commercial Street, London E1 6NF tel 0171 247 5385.

The Artist in the Changing City, 1nd edition, Williams, Bollen, Gidney & Owens, 1993, ISBN 09514763 1 9. Includes contacts list internationally for artists' workspaces. Price: £11.45 inc p&p .

British Council

Available from: British Council, 10 Spring Gardens, London SW1A 2BN

Studying Abroad, 1993. Leaflet briefly outlining schemes administered by the British Council and referring to other sources of information and publications. Price: free.

Charities Aid Foundation

Available from: Publications Department, Charities Aid Foundation, 48 Pembury Road, Tonbridge, Kent TN9 2JD

Directory of Grant-Making Trusts, 1993. Biannual, includes principle fields of interest of grant-making trusts in the UK; lists specific purpose and amounts of grants. Alphabetical register of grant-making organisations, with basic information. Usually available in major public and educational libraries. Price: £53.80 inc p&p.

Crafts Council

Available from: 44a Pentonville Road, London N1 9BY

Crafts Magazine. Broad-ranging magazine covering all aspects of contemporary craft practice.

Makers News. Sent free to makers on the Crafts Council slide index, details opportunities for craftspeople, emphasis on practical articles.

Croner Publications Ltd

Available from: 0181 547 3333

Croner's Reference Book for Exporters. The 'Bible ' for exporters, regularly updated. Notes for every country of the world, listing what paperwork is required and freight companies. Available in reference libraries.

Croner's Reference Book for the Self-Employed and Small Business. Loose-leaf book updated monthly with new information on legislation, regulations affecting the self-employed including exporting. Available in reference libraries.

Directory of Social Change

Available from: Directory of Social Change, Radius Works, Back Lane, London NW3 1HL. Postage £2.50 per order.

London Grants Guide, 2nd edition, ed. Lucy Stubbs, 1992, ISBN 0 907164 85 4. Covers grants for individuals and charities in London. Price: £12.50.

Major Companies Guide, ed. David Casson, 1994, ISBN 1 873860 22 6. Information on 400 major companies with policies, arts sponsorship and advice on applying. Price: £14.45 inc p&p.

DTI

Available from: Tel 0181 200 1992

Single Market, 1993. Set of publications including Guide to Sources of Advice and Europe Open to Professionals. Price: Free.

estamp

Available from: AN Publications (see above)

Europe for Printmakers, ed. Silvie Turner, 1993, ISBN 1 871831 08 3. An address notebook of printmaking networks throughout Europe. Large UK address section. Plus legal guide by Ros Innocent. Price: 12.95 inc p&p.

Eurofi plc

Available from: Guildgate House, Pelican Lane, Newbury RG13 1NX tel 01635 31900

Guide to European Union Grants & Loans. Comprehensive manual as a loose-leaf folder with update sheets. Price: £140 annual sub.

Europa Publications

International Foundation Directory, ed. Hodson, ISBN 09 46653 66 6. Annually published list of international charitable foundations. Usually available in main libraries. Price: £70.

European Commission.

Available from: Information Services Unit, Jean Monnet House, 8 Storey's Gate, London SW1P 3AT, tel: 0171 973 1992, fax: 0171 973 1900.

Europe in Your Area. Guide to local and regional contacts. Write or fax – the telephone queue can be interminable! Price: free.

Forlaget Scharff

Available from: AN Publications (see above)

Directory of International Open Art Exhibitions: Europe, ed. Judith Scharffenberg, 1993, ISBN 87 983852 0 8. Over 100 competitions and open exhibitions in Europe for painters, sculptors, printmakers, video artists and craftspeople with details of application and acceptance numbers, prices, deadlines and other valuable details. Covers up to 1998. Price: £12 inc p&p.

German Academic Exchange Service

Available from: German Academic Exchange Service (DAAD), 17 Bloomsbury Square, London WC1A 2LP, tel: 0171 404 4065.

Scholarships & Funding for Study & Research in Germany. Annual guide for British academic staff, researchers and students on their schemes and those offered by others, with eligibility and deadlines. Price: free.

H M Customs & Excise

Available from: HM Customs and Excise, New Kings Beam House, 22 Upper Ground, London SE1 9JP tel 0171 620 1313. See telephone directory for local office

ATA Carnets Europe Notice 756. Price: Free.

ATA Carnets, An International Customs Facilitation Scheme. Price: Free.

ATA Carnets Notice 104 Non-EC Countries. Issued by the Chamber of Commerce. Price: Free.

H M Customs & Excise Tariff. To be consulted in a reference library. Lists harmonised customs codes for goods.

Should I be registered for VAT? Form 700/1/91. Price: Free.

Health & Safety Commission

Information approved for the classification, packaging and labelling of dangerous substances for supply and conveyance by road, 2nd edition, 1988. Proper names and safety risks/ precautions of materials covered by Health & Safety regulations in the UK.

HMSO

Available from: HMSO bookshops and agents – see telephone directory.

Study Abroad – UNESCO, 1992, ISBN 923 00 27154. Biennial guide to grants and awards for overseas study. Price: £14.

Institute of International Education

Available from: 809 UN Plaza, New York, NY 10017, USA

Handbook on US Study for Foreign Nationals.

Specialised Study Options USA: A Guide to Short-Term Programs for Foreign Nationals Vol 1 Technical Programmes, Vol 2 Professional Development, ed. Marguerite Howard & Edrice Howard, 1986-1988.

Kelly' Export Services

Published each year with listings of all companies and sevices of interst to exporters. Consult in the public reference library.

Kogan Page

Available from: Kogan Page 120 Pentonville Rd, London N1 9JN, tel: 0171 278 0433.

Doing Business with the Japanese, John Abecasis-Phillips, 1992. A useful readable book described as "not a manual for doing business with the Japanese". Designed to help avoid some of the frustration often experienced by beginners Price: £14.95.

European Community Education Training and Research Programmes, ed. Preston, 1991, ISBN 0 7494 0438 8. Price: £22.50.

European Community Funding for Business Development, ed. European Policy Research Centre, 1993, ISBN 0 7494 0962 2. Guide to sources, grants and application procedures. Price: £50.

The Export Handbook, London Chamber of Commerce and Industry, 1993/4. Comprehensive book on EC regulations, planning an export strategy, overseas representation, documentation plus directory of suppliers of export services. May be available in public libraries. Price: £25.

Macmillan

The Grants Register. Lists research and project grants, scholarships and fellowships and exchange opportunities abroad primarily for postgraduate students. Usually available in main libraries.

National Council for Voluntary Organisations

Available from: National Council for Voluntary Organisations, Regent's Wharf, 8 All Saints Street, London N1 9RL tel 0171 713 6161.

Grants from Europe, Ann Davison & Bill Sealy, 1993, ISBN 0 71991304 7. Lists EC grants, gives advice on raising money and influencing policy. Not specifically for the arts. Price: £9.95.

Oxfam Publications

Available from: 274 Banbury Road, Oxford OX2 7DZ, tel: 01865 311311.

Export Marketing for a Small Handicraft Business, Edward Millard, 1992, ISBN 0 85598 174 1. Written for small businesses in the countries of the developing world who want to export craft goods to Europe. However, it offers sound business advice and export development strategy for small scale businesses and is worth consulting. Useful 'Ten Golden Rules' for the exporter. Price: £9.95 + £2 p&p.

PACT

Available from: PACT, Gordon House, 10 Greencoat Place, London SW1 1PH tel 0171 233 6000

Co-Production in Europe, Bertrand Moulier et al. Contact Janet Watson at PACT for further details. Price: £15 members, £30 otherwise.

Distribution and Exhibition, Shelly Bancroft. Outlines the process of distributing a film worldwide including possible deal structures, analysis of rights and territories and foreign distributors. Price: £10.

Prince's Trust

Available from: Central Books, 99 Wallis Road, London E9 5LN

Europe: A manual, 1992. Contacts and information sources in Europe, aimed at under 25 year olds but useful to others Price: £4.80 inc p&p.

Women Art Library

Available from: Women Art Library, Fulham Palace, Bishop's Avenue, London SW6 6EA tel 0171 731 7618

Women in the Arts – Networking Internationally, 1991, ISBN 0 7287 0632 6. Articles and information on international travel, exchange and opportunities for women, with international listing of women in the arts. Price: £3.

Women's Press

Available from: 34 Great Sutton Street, London EC1V 0DX

Europe: the Livewire guide to living and working in the EC. Aimed at young people but useful to others Price: £5.79 inc p&p.

Various business book on doing business in particular countries are published by the BBC, CBI and others. They can often be found in public libraries.

Index

Index

A growing series which reports on key aspects of contemporary visual arts practice. They combine analysis and commentary by visual arts experts with the thoughts and experiences of professional artists. Invaluable not only to artists, makers and photographers at all stages of their careers, art and design students, arts organisers, educationalists, careers and business advisers, but to all involved in promotion and development of the visual arts.

Art with People

Who is art for? Ever since community arts emerged in the '60s, there's been debate around this thorny question. And the arguments about process versus product, popular versus 'high' art and individual versus collective responsibility are as much aired now as they were then. *Art with People* traces the cultural and political aspirations of the early pioneers and sets them beside the environment for artists nowadays. By examining why artists choose to engage directly with people as animateurs, artists in residence and through community projects, the book shows how such working practices make the question "art for whom?" a millennium issue.

Chapters cover historical and contemporary context of community arts, artists' residencies, community initiatives, media-based projects and community education work. Writers include Sally Morgan, Felicity Allen, Esther Salamon, Suhail Khan, Sean Cubitt, and Nicholas Lowe. Artists and Groups featured include Open Hand Studios, Camerawork and Catalyst Arts, Alison Marchant and Ken Wolverton.
Ed. Malcolm Dickson, PB, A5, 136pp, illus, ISBN 0 907730 23 X, £7.25

Artists' Stories

What do visual artists do? Paint pictures, design seats, have families, run galleries, construct bridges, shoot films, make sculpture, get into debt, travel the world. A 'career' can mean doing many different things at the same time, involve radical changes of direction and be interrupted by personal circumstances. Keeping work going may often not be easy or remunerative. In *Artists' Stories* up-and-coming and well-established artists, makers and photographers describe how it's worked out for them. Aimed at art and design students, recent graduates and arts educationalists, this book also deserves to be read by all involved in the development of visual arts.

Features 24 artists including Richard La Trobe-Bateman, Lei Cox, John Darwell, Hilary Green, Jane Hamlyn, Karen Knorr, Mary O'Mahony and Janice Tchalenko, Mike Stubbs.
Anna Douglas, Nick Wegner, PB, A4, 80pp, illus, ISBN 0 9077 24 8, £7.25

Investigating Galleries
the artist's guide to exhibiting

The question of how to get work seen by more than the cat and the gasman is answered in this book. Full of information and strategies to improve an artist's chance of exhibiting and minimise the risk of rejection and discouragement, it explains why artists need to investigate their own self-image, ambitions and long-term aspirations and have a clear understanding of how the art world operates before they embark on an exhibiting career. Sound advice on approaching galleries and presenting work, on sales commission, promotion and gallery education strategies means that artists who are young or isolated will find this book invaluable, and the more experienced will discover it inspires new approaches and a sharper plan of action.
Debbie Duffin, PB, A5, 120pp, illus, ISBN 0 907730 22 1, £7.25

Organising Your Exhibition

Full of sound, practical advice on all aspects of exhibition organisation and an ideal companion to Investigating Galleries, it offers an instant solution to the agonies of organising a show. Covering everything from showing in alternative spaces to the tools needed to get a show up and from how to locate spaces and selling the work, it even tells you how to estimate the wine needed for the private view!
Debbie Duffin, PB, A5, 116pp, ISBN 0 907730 14 0, £7.25

Making Ways

the visual artists' guide to surviving and thriving

Quite apart from helping artists, makers and photographers to grapple with the loathsome necessities of exhibiting, selling, self-employment, planning work, etc, this book offers plenty of sound, witty and inspiring advice on how to actually thrive. As well as covering the myriad of ways visual artists can get involved in community-based work, it also has chapters on health and safety, benefits, copyright and financial administration. There is little that practitioners need to know which isn't included here.
Ed. David Butler, PB, A5, 256pp, illus, ISBN 0 907730 16 7, £11.99

Art in Public

what, why and how

An intelligent guide to the complex theoretical and practical issues affecting art in public, a field of work which includes both the infamous 'turd in the plaza' and the genuinely popular and imaginative initiatives which transform and revitalise public spaces. Art in Public provides a thought-provoking account of the values and philosophies which give rise to the range work and debates their implications for art, the artist and the public. Commissioners, agencies and artist have found this an invaluable reference, and even artists, makers and photographers with no intention of 'going public' at present will find this a stimulating introduction to debate which is set to run and run.
Ed. Susan Jones, PB, 178pp, illus, ISBN 0 907730 18 3, £9.95

Fundraising

Genuinely qualifies for the 'indispensable' tag, this book describes the range of possibilities for artists, makers and photographers to finance exhibitions, projects, travel and workspaces. Excellent sections on developing a strategy and making proposals along with revealing comments from those on the receiving-end of applications make this a recommended book not only for individual artists but for groups and small organisations involved in developing projects with artists.
Ed. Susan Jones, PB, A5, 134pp, illus, ISBN 0 907730 20 5, £7.25

Selling

This should be compulsory reading for those artists who believe that if left to its own devices in studio, gallery or on top of the wardrobe, work will somehow contrive to sell itself. Selling examines the ins and outs of selling and illustrates how artists, makers and photographers have benefited from a more pro-active approach. It explains how to work out prices and identify the best outlets, and looks in detail at the advantages and disadvantages of everything from trade fairs and agents to exhibitions and commissions.
Judith Staines, PB, A5, 136pp, Illus, ISBN 0 907730 19 1, £7.25

Directory of Exhibition Spaces

Seeking to show? Fixing an exhibition tour? The Directory of Exhibition Spaces covers everything you need to know about galleries showing temporary programmes of contemporary visual arts, crafts, photography and live art performances. It lists over 2100 galleries and exhibition spaces – however large or small – in the UK and Ireland, describing art forms shown, exhibition policy and gallery space. Also includes access information for disabled visitors. To make it user-friendly for artists, exhibition organisers and visual arts professionals the directory has been indexed by arts funding region/county/ town as well as by gallery highlighting art forms shown, if applications are welcome and whether space is hired out.
Ed. Janet Ross, published end of JUNE 95, PB, 336pp, ISBN 0 907730 27 2, £13.99.

Artist Handbooks

Live Art

Designed for all visual artists whose work involves live or temporary activities, *Live Art* combines information about the aspirations and experiences of artists with the practical considerations of putting on an event. A useful guide for artists, promoters and curators.
Ed. Robert Ayers & David Butler, PB, A5, 178pp, illus, ISBN 0 907730 13 2, £7.25

Across Europe

the artist's guide to travel and work

Looks at 24 European countries through the eyes of artists who live there and UK artists who've lived, studied or worked there and in doing so, provides valuable insights into each country's cultural character and the practicalities of exhibiting, selling, creating opportunities and making contacts. Comes with a free copy of the *Artists & the EU* Fact Pack (worth £1.85) which covers artists' rights and responsibilities, sources of information and advice, and gives profiles of EU countries.
Ed. David Butler, PB, A5, 168pp, illus, ISBN 0 907730 15 9, £9.95

Money Matters

Problems with pricing? Baffled by book-keeping? Get Money Matters: the artist's financial guide and stop the headaches. Changes in how tax is calculated for self-employed people, and the introduction of self-assessment (working out your own tax bill) make it more important than ever for people running small businesses to have a good grasp of financial systems. This fully-revised second edition provides expert advice on taxation and the Inland Revenue, National Insurance, VAT, pricing work, and handling customers, suppliers and banks. And all this is backed-up with a model accounting system written especially for visual arts and crafts businesses.
Richard Murphy, Sarah Deeks & Sally Nolan, PB, 134pp, ISBN 0 907730 26 4, £7.25

Copyright

Expert advice about the applications of the 1988 Copyright, Designs & Patents Act, negotiating agreements, making sure you get the best from selling your copyright and how to deal with infringements. Contains practical examples of how artists, makers and photographers have dealt with copyright and reproduction issues.
Roland Miller, PB, A5, 125pp, illus, ISBN 0 907730 12 4, £7.25

Artists Newsletter

The monthly magazine providing analysis, commentary and information across contemporary visual arts practice.

ARTISTS & ARTWORK features review-based articles by curators, critics and artists commenting on what lies behind current practice. It covers exhibitions, installations, art in public, new media and issue-based projects. OUTLOOK is an illustrated round-up of new work, and WHAT'S ON is the monthly guide to temporary exhibitions and live art events around the country.

The **PRACTICAL PAGES** give comprehensive information on opportunities across the visual arts. Over 1000 are listed each year, including open exhibitions, gallery calls for applications, awards, residencies, commissions, mail-art, art and craft fairs and competitions. Features providing expert technical and business advice are run alongside the Help page, Small Ads, Sits Vac and the artists' contact page Pinboard.

In **ISSUES AND NEWS,** writers from the world of arts, education and politics map out the social, economic and political context for the arts, and in-depth articles are linked with short reports on issues.

Twelve issues a year, available from selected retail outlets at £2 a copy, or by mail-order subscription.

Individual ■ UK £19.95
■ Europe £28
■ Overseas £36

Institution ■ UK, Europe, Overseas £36

Prices quoted as at May 1995 are subject to alteration, please check before ordering.

Visual Arts Contracts

an

Introduction to Contracts

Designed to be read as the first step to making professional legal agreements, *Introduction to Contracts,* outlines the elements and terms you might find in a contract, and provides artists with the ammunition they need to negotiate, deal with disputes and find a suitable solicitor.

PB, A4, 12pp, £1.50

Residencies

Demystifies the legal arrangements for artists' residencies in any kind of settings. The ready-to-use contract form for a residency deals with having more than one partner in an agreement, and the workshop contract can be adapted for many 'one-off' activities. Also contains notes on employment and tax, copyright, moral and reproduction rights.

PB, A4, 20pp, ISBN 0 907730 25 6, £3.50

Commission Contracts

Maps out the legal arrangements necessary for all those who work with commissions and public art. By comparing public and private arrangements and describing the roles of parties in public art commissions, functions of agents and dealers and the implications of sub-contracting. Fill-in contract forms for Commissioned Design, Commission and Sale for Public Art and Private Commission Contract.

PB, A4, 20pp, £3.50

Licensing Reproductions

Make the most of your images by getting the licensing agreements right. This contract sets out how to grant or obtain permission to reproduce artwork or designs, and includes details of what licensing agreements to use, and notes on fees and royalties and negotiating and monitoring agreements.

PB, A4, 20pp, £3.50

NAA Public Exhibition Contract

The National Artists Association, commissioned this contract to cover the legal arrangements surrounding showing work in public galleries and exhibition spaces. Many artists, makers and photographers as well as galleries have found it an invaluable way to clarify responsibilities. It includes ready-to-use contract forms for a public exhibition and an exhibition tour, along with information on fees, selling, insurance and promotion.

PB, A4, 24pp, £3.50

Selling Contracts

If selling is part of your practice, then you need this contract. It deals exclusively with selling art and craft work and covers selling to private buyers, galleries and shops, and includes a contract form for selling on sale or return.

PB, A4, 14pp, £3.50

Ordering details

For mail orders add £1.50 per order for postage (UK), £2.50 per order (Europe), £4 per order (Overseas). Telephone credit card orders to 0191 514 3600 (Ref EI), or write to: AN Publications, PO Box 23, Sunderland SR4 6DG (prices quoted at May '95 are subject to change, please check before ordering).

Developed because the visual arts profession needed effective agreements to cover all aspects of contemporary visual arts prac- tice, our Visual Arts Contracts will ensure that collab- orations between artists, exhibition organisers, agents, and commission- ers are profession- al and harmonious. Written by Nicholas Sharp – a solicitor specialis- ing in contract preparation and negotiation for business and the arts – they are legally sound, and contain either ready-to-fill-in forms or a point- by-point checklist with explanatory notes. Each comes with per- mission for the purchaser to make additional copies for their own pro- fessional use.

Help us to improve our books

...help us stay in touch with your needs and interests by filling in and returning this freepost form. Your opinions are important and will help us to continue to publish the kinds of books you need, when you need them. To thank you for your help, we will send you a £2 discount voucher for use when purchasing other books from AN Publications.

Title of book

Where did you buy it?

Why did you choose it?

☐ Best coverage of the subject   ☐ Recognised the author

☐ Recognised the publisher   ☐ Well priced

☐ Other (please specify)

Where did you hear about this book?

☐ Book review in

☐ Leaflet in

☐ Advertisment in

☐ Browsing in   bookshop

☐ Personal recommendation

☐ Other (please specify)

Have you any comments on the content of this book?

Name   Address

Postcode   Tel

Send to: **Julie Crawshaw, AN Publications, Freepost, PO Box 23, Sunderland, SR1 1BR, tel 0191 567 3589, fax 0191 564 1600.**   Ref OR